TONED ARMS
IN TEN DAYS

TONED ARMS
IN TEN DAYS

MATTHEW GRACE

with Laura Tucker

BERKLEY BOOKS, NEW YORK

TONED ARMS IN TEN DAYS

A Berkley Book / published by arrangement with
LifeTime Media, Inc.

NOTE: Every effort has been made to ensure that the information contained in this book is complete and accurate. However, neither the publisher, packager nor the author is engaged in rendering professional advice or services to the individual reader. The ideas, procedures, and suggestions contained in this book are not intended as a substitute for consulting with your physician. All matters regarding your health require medical supervision. Neither the author, packager nor the publisher shall be liable or responsible for any loss, injury, or damage allegedly arising from any information or suggestion in this book. The opinions expressed in this book represent the personal views of the author and not of the publisher.

PRINTING HISTORY
Berkley edition / May 2003

Copyright © 2003 by LifeTime Media, Inc.
Book design by Julie Rogers
Interior illustrations by Linda Parker Crank
Cover design by Lesley Worrell
Cover photograph by RNT Productions/Corbis

For information address: The Berkley Publishing Group,
a division of Penguin Group (USA) Inc.,
375 Hudson Street, New York, New York 10014.

ISBN: 0-425-19112-5

BERKLEY®
Berkley Books are published by The Berkley Publishing Group,
a division of Penguin Group (USA) Inc.,
375 Hudson Street, New York, New York 10014.
BERKLEY and the "B" design
are trademarks belonging to Penguin Group (USA) Inc.

PRINTED IN THE UNITED STATES OF AMERICA

10 9 8 7 6 5 4 3 2 1

CONTENTS

chapter one

THE TONED ARMS OF YOUR DREAMS

ARE YOU REALLY happy with the way you look in a strapless dress? Or do you walk by racks of sleeveless tops without even stopping to look? Do you automatically throw a shirt over your tank top before you leave the house? Do your upper arms look strong, toned, and sculpted, or is there a little more jiggle and wiggle in that area than you'd like others to see?

I've been a private personal trainer in Manhattan for fifteen years, and I've worked with all kinds of people, of varying levels of fitness. I've also worked with a number of celebrities who have needed, for various professional reasons, to get into really great shape in only a short period of time. I devised this program, Toned Arms in Ten Days, to help people like them, who want to get into shape *fast*.

It can work for you, too. Whether you're someone who just wants to wear something a little more daring to a special event, a bride with a short amount of time before the big day, or you just want to get in better shape, this book is your ticket to beautiful arms. This book also offers the perfect opportunity for those of you who have gotten away from your workout routine or fallen into a fitness rut, and would like to kick your program into a slightly higher gear in order to see some immediate results.

The actual ten-day program is very simple. It requires that you do three, easy-to-learn exercises, which I call the Basics. If you do three to five rounds of the Basics every day for ten days, you will see results. If you alter your diet according to my nutritional suggestions and add the aerobic workout, you'll see great results.

For those of you with a slightly higher level of fitness commitment, I've also included three other sets of exercises that you can add on to your basic workout. You'll still be doing the Basics every day, but you'll also be adding two or three sets of these extra exercises. These work slightly different parts of the major muscle groups in the arms, and in different ways. Adding the additional programs—in the sequence in which I've given them—will refine your workout slightly, and keep you on your toes. Once you've been working out for a while, you'll know which exercises work best for you, and you can mix and match your own rounds.

I've also included a chapter specifically for the advanced beginner, so it'll be a while before you outgrow this book!

I've dedicated my life to physical fitness, and I think it's an essential part of a balanced lifestyle. I'm certainly not recommending that you do this program for ten days and then quit! I like to think of this ten-day program as a way to start a weight-training and exercise regimen. I think that when you see the change in the way you look and feel after you've been working out for ten days, you're going to have all the motivation you need to keep going. With that in mind, I've outlined a plan that will allow you to turn your ten-day workout into a maintenance workout that you can incorporate into your life—indefinitely.

Nothing motivates like results. It's going to be a lot easier to pass up that ice cream when you see how great you look in your new sleeveless top. I know you're going to be amazed when you see how much control you have over the way your body looks and feels, and I predict that you'll feel the impact of those changes in all areas of your life. Who doesn't want to feel stronger, firmer, more confident, more attractive? Isn't it time you made a commitment to your good health? Since results are so easily obtainable when you train with weights, congratulations are in order—you're on the brink of a healthy revolution!

chapter two

EXPLODING THE MYTHS

THERE ARE SO many myths surrounding women and weight lifting that I thought we'd go through some of them and see what's really going on. As far as I'm concerned, all these myths do is prevent women from looking their best. (You'll notice that I'm being charitable and calling them "myths" instead of "lies" or "excuses." All the same, you should feel free to come back and read this chapter if you find yourself invoking one of these "myths" in order to get out of a workout.)

MYTH: IF I LIFT WEIGHTS, I'LL GET HUGE "MAN ARMS."
This is probably the most common argument I hear against weight lifting—even from some of the female clients I work with—and I'm always surprised by it.

All I have to say is: If only it were that easy. There's no way that you're going to get huge, Popeye-on-spinach arms all of a sudden without a genie's intervention. It's just not going to happen. Building muscles is a gradual process, and while you should notice an immediate difference in the way your body looks, major changes will only happen gradually.

In this program, you're not going to be *bodybuilding,* you're going to be *weight training*. These are two totally different animals! In bodybuilding, you move a lot of weight for a few repetitions. Our focus, on the other hand, is on strengthening and lengthening your muscles, not on adding a huge amount of bulky mass to your frame. For this reason, I do not recommend that you ever use dumbbells weighing more than fifteen pounds.

This is not to say that you can't get too muscular or too defined, although it's hard to imagine this happening without you being aware of it. If you do find that you want a more feminine look to your arms, all you need to do is scale back your upper-arm training. In fact, the whole point of this book is to show you that you're in control of this process.

Not only can you get in shape, but you can control the *kind* of shape you achieve by changing the way you train. That goes for toning down as well as toning up.

I can guarantee that it'll take you a long time and a lot of work to get those huge, seam-splitting arms you're so afraid of. In the unlikely event that it does happen, by that point you'll be well educated about your own body and how to train and will easily be able to make a correction. You're going to become your own sculptor. Your body is the clay.

There's another myth, sort of the opposite to the "man arms" one, and it goes something like this: Women *can't* gain muscle because they lack sufficient testosterone or some other nonsense. I'm not even going to bother debunking that one. Work out for ten days and debunk it yourself.

MYTH: IF I STOP TRAINING, ALL THE MUSCLE I'VE GAINED WILL TURN INTO FAT.

This one drives me nuts, too! Fat cells and muscle cells are completely different. Muscle does not and cannot turn into fat. Period. End of story. If you stop training, you will eventually lose muscle tone and definition, but that muscle *never* becomes fat regardless of how it appears.

The good news is that lost muscle is easier to

regain than muscle that was never developed to begin with. In other words, it will be easier for you to get back in shape if you've dropped off for a little while.

MYTH: WEIGHT TRAINING WILL MAKE ME STIFF, DECREASING MY FLEXIBILITY.

A lot of people believe that weight training will make them tight and stiff, and this belief is emphasized by the soreness felt whenever anyone begins a new exercise program. In fact, the exact opposite is true. If you do these exercises properly (and I can't emphasize the word *properly* enough), you'll find that your flexibility *increases*.

Soreness *is* a part of weight training when you're just starting out. When you train, you change your body, and what you're feeling is that change. Actually, what you're feeling is a buildup of lactic acid, but the result of that buildup is a changed muscle (we'll talk more about how the whole thing works later).

There's a big difference between soreness and pain. Pain comes when you've injured yourself by exercising too hard or with incorrect form. I'll say this again, but hear me now: If something you're doing hurts, or if you ever feel a sharp stabbing pain, you should stop *immediately*. Soreness and muscle burn are something else entirely. I personally love the slight feeling of soreness that comes the day after I've really pushed myself past my limits. It's like a souvenir that I get to carry around with me for a little while, a badge of honor, and a physical marker of how good it felt to push my body past what it's used to doing. You'll grow to love the feeling, too. Wear your soreness with pride!

Bear in mind that the best way to get rid of soreness is to simply work out again! You'll notice that stiffness going away by the second or third set. Sometimes, particularly if you've trained hard the day before, you'll notice that you're having more difficulty than usual working those same muscles. That's great! It means that you're in the process of changing the muscle. Don't worry—you're not getting weaker, you're just working tired muscles. The work you're doing counts anyway, even if those reps don't feel like they're coming as easily. Don't ever drop back to a lower weight class. If you have to do fewer reps or take a five-second break before you can continue, that's fine. Don't get discouraged, and you'll soon see that you've surpassed your own limits again and again.

MYTH: WEIGHT TRAINING WILL MAKE ME TIRED.

If you're burning more energy in your workouts, you'll have less energy for your life, right?

It's easy to see why this is such a common belief, but it ignores the basic mechanics of the way the body works. The fact is that people who are fit have *more* energy, not less. Their bodies work better because they're more efficient machines.

When you work out with weights, not only will your arms start to look fantastic, but they'll also work better. That's because the muscles you're building are muscles you need in everyday life, and when you build them, you increase your functional strength. After you've been training for a while, you'll discover that it's not only easier to lift that ten-pound dumbbell than it used to be, but it'll also be easier to lift the other stuff in your life, like groceries and toddlers and UPS packages. One of my clients, a busy attorney, was amazed to discover after a couple of weeks that her ordinarily cumbersome briefcase was starting to feel feather-light, even after a long day at court.

It's also important to remember that along with getting stronger, you'll also be increasing the efficiency of your heart and lungs. If your heart and lungs are out of shape, everything is difficult—walking up a couple of flights of stairs can put you out of commission for the rest of the day. But if you're in good shape, getting to the third floor takes a lot less out of you, and you have more energy left over for the rest of your life.

That said, many people do notice a slight sag in their energy level when they start training. It takes a good deal of energy to change your body! Take care of yourself. Get lots of sleep, eat good food, and I promise that you'll feel better, especially when you start seeing the way your new body looks in the mirror! If you stick with the program, I guarantee that you'll have much more energy for your life.

MYTH: I'M TOO WEAK TO LIFT WEIGHTS.

You may have very little upper-body strength right now. That's okay! It's certainly no reason not to train.

It doesn't matter where you start, as long as you start. Dumbbells are available in very light weight classes, as low as a single pound. This isn't a competition—as you'll see when we get into the specific exercises, it's essential to choose a weight you can handle so that you can complete the exercise without losing your form. If that's a one- or two-pound dumbbell, then that's what you'll use.

Almost everyone can lift some weight, and I recommend that you try a one-pound weight, or even a roll of quarters to start. I have worked with a few people who really were too weak to lift weights, especially people coming back from serious injuries or illness. In those cases, we simply didn't use weights at all. You can do all the exercises I've provided here without weights, and your body will provide a nàtural resistance. It took a very short amount of time—no more than a week—to get these people's muscles (and minds) in good enough condition to start using weights. If you follow the program and do the exercises without weights, you'll soon see an improvement in your body and will build your strength to the point where you need weights to continue to improve. That can be one of your goals.

MYTH: I HAVE AN INJURY, AND WORRY THAT I'LL HURT MYSELF AGAIN.

Many dancers and professional athletes recovering from sports-related injuries have discovered that weight training can do for them what massage and ultrasound had failed to accomplish. In fact, weight training is incorporated into most rehabilitative physical therapy programs because of its proven effectiveness in rebuilding healthy muscle and improving circulation.

I had a client, a former professional ballerina, who had come out of retirement to dance on Broadway. Although the work for the show was considerably less demanding than what she had been used to, she found herself suffering from chronic and debilitating back pain. We started slowly, but after two and a half weeks of weight training, she was noticeably better, and after a month, she experienced a complete recovery, something she was unable to get from doctors. We had strengthened her supporting muscles so that her poor back didn't have to do all the work.

When you start to lift weights after recovery, keep the weights light at first, and stop immediately if there's any sharp pain. If you are unable to extend (stretch) and flex the muscle you wish to work without experiencing severe pain, you need to wait until you get a full range of motion back. Only you can know when you are ready for added resistance, but a physical therapist can certainly aid you in this decision.

Again, if you're recovering from a serious injury, it's totally acceptable to do the program without any weights at all for the first week. You will gain some strength and flexibility just by using your own body weight for resistance.

Proper weight training will increase your overall strength and flexibility, and can help injured tissues rebuild and revitalize. If you're concerned, talk to your orthopedist or physical therapist before you start working out. Show them the exercises that you're planning to do, and ask if they can suggest modifications, if needed. Remember, resistance training is a real confidence builder, and confidence is one of the most important (and most neglected) aspects of recovering from a physical injury. Resistance training teaches us to trust our bodies again, and to feel confident about our strength and skill, and it gives us easily measured results to take pride in. For that reason alone, it's a wonderful form of physical therapy.

MYTH: I NEED TO LOSE WEIGHT, SO I NEED AEROBICS MORE THAN I NEED WEIGHT TRAINING.

It's true that the two most effective ways to lose weight are to eat better and to do cardiovascular exercise. I do recommend that everyone do some kind of low-impact cardiovascular exercise for at least half an hour, three to five times a week.

What a lot of people don't know is that resistance training can *be* cardiovascular exercise. Best of all, it's low-impact cardiovascular training, unlike running or dance aerobics, which means that it's better for your joints. It's the most efficient way to exercise out there: if you do the program I've set out here, and you do the exercises in the order I suggest with little or no rest between them, you will reap cardiovascular benefits, and you will lose weight.

When you train regularly, your metabolism will speed up. Your circulation will increase, so your body will hold more oxygen. Your digestive system will work better. Your skin will look more healthy and youthful. And as your musculature improves, you'll burn more calories, because muscular people burn more calories when they're resting than less muscular people do.

You'll look much better after training, even if you didn't lose a single pound. Trust me: 140 pounds of well-toned muscle looks a lot better than 140 pounds of flab. And if you go from 140 pounds of flab to 120 pounds of well-toned muscle, you're going to be very happy with the results.

Don't let yourself use these myths as excuses, and don't let other people tell you differently. Bookmark this chapter, and if you find yourself confronted by some of these myths in action, feel free to quote me. Or you can just let your fabulous new arms speak for themselves.

chapter three

RECIPE FOR A HEALTHIER LIFE:
THE BENEFITS OF WEIGHT TRAINING

GETTING IN SHAPE through resistance weight training is one of the most positive changes you can make in your life. Whether you're using this ten-day program to get ready for an event, or to kick-start a major lifestyle and fitness overhaul, you'll notice a positive improvement in your health and overall well-being.

After you've been training for a while, your circulation will improve, and your eyes and complexion will look clearer and brighter. Your aches and pains will melt away, and you'll notice increased flexibility and strength. You'll lift your five-year-old easily out of the pool, without feeling like your arms are being ripped out of their sockets, and you won't get winded walking up stairs. Your cholesterol may be lower during your next physical, and your bone density and strength will increase as well.

Weight training also gives the body a better overall shape. I know that many women spend a lot of time at the gym on the treadmill, StairMaster, and elliptical trainer. Outside of the gym, they walk and make sure to take the stairs. I certainly don't discourage this kind of muscle-building cardiovascular exercise, because it's really good for you, but it's not the only thing you need to do to look and feel good.

All the exercises I mentioned before have one thing in common: they work the lower half of the body. If you're not working out your upper body as well, the body you're building is going to look uneven. I hear so many women complaining about their "pear" shape—narrow shoulders combined with wide hips and thighs. When all your major training work is going on below the waist, you're just encouraging that pear. A little work on the upper body does an enormous amount to even out your shape and give a sense of balance to the entire body.

When you resistance-train, you're not only working all the major muscles, you're also working the network of smaller supporting muscles that control your every move. So don't be surprised if you notice that you're moving with more grace and control, and that your reflexes have improved. Your body will look better. Your clothes will fit you better—or you'll find you need new ones altogether. You'll discover gorgeous, taut planes and curves in places where there was once nothing but flab and jiggle.

Weight and resistance training will make you feel better, too. It's a well-documented fact that working out with weights increases the number of endorphins, the "happy" chemicals, released by your brain. And when you see how terrific you look with your new toned arms, you'll be even happier! We feel better about ourselves when we look better, and we feel even better when we've proven, to ourselves and to others, that we have the discipline and motivation to get those results.

Obviously, I believe that resistance training is an essential ingredient in an overall fitness regimen. It may also surprise you to hear that I believe it's an essential ingredient in a healthy life. I often tell my clients that "You live the way you train, and you train the way you live."

What does this mean? Well, you can learn a lot about yourself from the way you work out. As you start training, notice your internal reactions to the challenges that you encounter. Is it hard for you to maintain concentration? How do you react when you encounter difficulty? Do you quit as soon as the going gets tough? Do you fade at the end of an exercise, letting your posture and form get sloppy? Do you fail to follow through? Is your tendency to rest on your laurels, instead of noting your progress and redoubling your efforts to see even better results?

We often encounter difficulties in our lives, and our instinct is to shrink, to quit, to change our course. The same thing often happens when we work out. When it gets hard and we begin to experience discomfort, we either stop the exercise or we let our form fall apart, taking the intensity off the muscle we're working. How many great ideas never see the light of day because someone got discouraged by repeated rejections and quit? How many failed businesses might have succeeded if the principals had stuck to good form instead of taking shortcuts and cheating when the road got bumpy?

The good news is that you can use your workouts as a laboratory for change in your life. "Living the way you train" is more than a metaphor. If you bring mindfulness and discipline and self-respect to your workout, you can't help but bring it into the rest of your life as well. If you can teach yourself to stay in the moment while you're at the gym (or your living room, backyard, or wherever you work out), you will bring that ability into the rest of your life. If you can teach yourself to keep working past the burn in your biceps in order to see results, you will be better able to survive discomfort and pain in your life at large. If you honor yourself by sticking with a program that will make for a better, stronger you, you'll be more dedicated to finding the best possible version of yourself in everything that you do.

chapter four

HOW YOUR MUSCLES WORK

MOST OF US don't think too much about how our
bodies work. But if you're going to change your
body, it will help if you understand a little about how
the whole process works.

Here's something to think about: No matter how
unfit you look and feel right now, all the muscles
you're ever going to have are already there. No matter how hard you work out, you're not actually going
to build any new muscles, you're just going to
improve the ones you already have.

More good news: The more out of shape you are,
the faster you're going to see results, and the more
dramatic those results are going to be. The better

condition a muscle is in, the harder it is to affect it—it's just one of the paradoxes of weight training. So the fitter you get, the harder you'll have to work to improve . . . but let's cross that bridge when we come to it.

I'll be honest with you. If you are more than twenty pounds over your ideal body weight, it is going to be difficult to get your "dream arms" in just ten days. Because of the fat between the muscle and the skin, the shape and definition of the muscle will be lost. That does not mean you can't make dramatic changes in your arms or your overall physical condition in the next ten days. It just means you're going to have to take incremental steps toward your goal, and broaden your timeframe by a few weeks.

If you're overweight, the only way to look toned is to actually lose weight. You know those big bouncer guys, who have what a friend of mine calls "the Biker Body"? Those guys just look fat—until you hit them, and then you realize that there's a pretty solid layer of muscle underneath there. The only thing separating their bodies from the ripped bodies that you see at Muscle Beach is a layer of fat. You can be a really muscular person, but you're not going to look cut and toned until you've gotten rid of the fat that covers those muscles.

After losing the fat, muscle tone really is the key

to looking good. We've all seen skinny people without any muscle tone—and it's clearly not the answer. Losing fat without adding muscle tone doesn't look healthy either.

If you weight-train correctly, with only minimal rests between exercise sets as I will explain later, you'll start eliminating the layer of flab that's hiding those muscles from the world. You'll be getting the best of both worlds: you're burning fat while you're building muscle. If you're also eating better, you're going to start to see weight loss without even really trying.

THE ARM

Let's take a look at the body part in question: your arm.

Like all our limbs, the arm is made up of a number of different muscles. One of the common training mistakes is to work one muscle heavily and neglect the others. Great arms are *balanced* arms—it's imperative that you give each muscle group in the arm equal attention (and do the same regimen for both arms).

What are these different muscle groups?

The three major ones that we'll be dealing with in the toned-arms workout are the deltoid (the shoulder muscle), the biceps (the muscle on the front of the upper arm), and the triceps (the muscle at the back of the upper arm). It's unlikely you'll have a toned arm without working all of them.

Note: These are all upper-arm muscles. The forearm, which is the big muscle in the lower arm, is the other major muscle in the arm, but since most of the women I've encountered are predominantly worried about improving their upper arms, and since many of the exercises presented here also work the forearms, we're going to concentrate on the deltoid, triceps, and biceps.

THE SHOULDER

You know where your shoulder is, but did you know the muscles it contains are among the most important in your body? Many people don't, and they tend to neglect the shoulders in their workouts.

Working the shoulder muscle is crucial if you want to have a well-balanced arm. It's also a way to make your whole body look better. One of the primary causes of poor posture is inadequate shoulder strength. When your shoulders are rounded and stooped, you look shorter, older, and less fit than you are, and you can suffer serious back and neck problems as a result. Plus, women gain weight easily in their hips and thighs, and those are the areas they tend to work out most as well. What better way to even out a pear-shaped body than to widen and sculpt the shoulders to improve your overall proportions.

THE TRICEPS

You know that jiggle underneath the back of your arm? That muscle (or the muscle that's hiding under the fat) is the triceps.

Flabby triceps are probably the most common reason why women feel self-conscious in sleeveless dresses and tank tops. Unless you specifically address these muscles, they don't get better as you get older, although a lot of women tell me that they've never felt confident about this part of their bodies.

Well, all that's going to change, starting now.

THE BICEPS

This is the muscle that bulges when Popeye eats spinach. Make a fist, raise your arm, squeeze like a bodybuilder—and whatever pops out is your biceps. Less than impressed? Don't worry. It's one of the easiest muscles in the body to build, and a sculpted biceps will make an enormous difference in the way your arm looks (and works!).

RESISTANCE TRAINING

Now we know the muscles we're dealing with, let's look at how they actually work. Here are the basics: Muscles are attached to bones. When your brain sends electrical messages to the muscles, telling them to move, the fibers contract or lengthen, pulling the bone they're attached to like a lever.

Muscles come in opposing pairs—one to pull the bone one way, one to push it another. When one of these muscles is contracted, or shortened, the opposing muscle is usually relaxed, or lengthened. Let's look at an example, and you can use your own arm as a study guide if you'd like. The triceps and the biceps are opposing muscles. Bend your arm, bringing your fist toward you, making that bodybuilder muscle we talked about before. You're contracting your biceps muscle, and it's pulling the bone of your lower arm along with it. Do you see how that contraction shortens the biceps muscle and stretches the triceps? When you straighten the arm, the triceps is shortened, and the biceps lengthens.

In order to get the maximum benefit from weight training, we have to work during both cycles: while the muscle is lengthening as well as when it's shortening. Concentric contraction is what it's called when the muscle shortens. Eccentric contraction is when the muscle lengthens. Isometric contraction involves contraction but no movement in the joint.

(Put your hand against the wall and push as hard as you can—that's an isometric contraction.)

When you curl your biceps during one of our basic exercises, that's concentric contraction at work. When you release the weight back to the ready position, that's eccentric contraction. There's a tendency to get sloppy, letting the weight drop down during the second part of the exercise, so that you're letting gravity do the work for you. When you do that, you're just wasting time and cheating yourself. If you want to see results, you'll slow it down, controlling the movement of the weight the whole way down. That way, you're working what we call the "negative" contraction, the eccentric contraction, as hard as you work the concentric one. You're getting twice the work done in the same amount of time. Two for the price of one!

And, as you'll see, sometimes I'll have you hold the weight at the top of the exercise for a second or two. That's an isometric contraction, so you're actually working all three phases of muscle contraction when you're training correctly. The bargain keeps getting better!

The human body is an awesome machine, and one of the things it's best at is healing muscle. When muscles are damaged, they heal themselves so well that they're better than they were before—they come back stronger and fitter every time. What you're doing when you weight-train is safely "overworking" those muscles so that they can heal better than they were.

Whenever your muscle pushes or pulls against a force, it has to work harder than usual to contract. The amount of force that the muscle is contracting against and the number of times it does so are the factors that make a muscle fitter, and therefore "better" at contracting. So your muscles need something to work against in order for them to get stronger. That's where the idea of resistance comes in. Weights, in the form of dumbbells, are the primary form of resistance we use in the toned-arms workout, although you will be using your own body weight as resistance when we get to push-ups as well.

In order to make your muscles stronger, you have to push them a little. In fitness parlance, this is called muscle overload, which sounds worse than it really is. All it means is that you have to work the muscle to the point of fatigue—and a little bit past it—to see results. You can tell your muscle is beginning to get overloaded when you start to feel the infamous "burn." As your muscles produce energy, they produce an overage of lactic acid, which changes the acidity level of the cells. That's the burn you feel.

It's typical for people to want to quit when they start to feel the burning in the muscle, but that will slow your progress. I like to think of that burning sensation as the *beginning* of the toning, instead of the end of it. Every repetition that you do before the burn is little more than maintenance—but every rep you do *after* you start to feel that burn means that you are forcing the muscle to change, and that's golden.

Eventually, you won't be able to complete another rep. Your form will start to fall apart as your arm gets heavier and heavier, and you may feel the muscles begin to shake. This is called failure, but it actually means the exact opposite! *Failure means you've successfully overloaded the arm.* You have to work to failure every time you work the muscle, or you're not getting the best workout you can. This is why it's so important—and efficient—to concentrate as much on those negative reps as on the primary movement. The faster you fatigue the muscle, and the longer you work the fatigued muscle—the more slow reps you can squeeze out of your tired arms before failing completely—the faster you'll start to see results.

As you get stronger, that point of fatigue will change. You'll find yourself cranking out sets of biceps curls with weights that you could hardly lift once when you started. That's terrific, but whipping through a once-difficult workout is not going to make you stronger. As your muscle condition improves, you have to increase the resistance and/or the number of reps and sets per workout. *To see results, you have*

Exercise Terms

In order to avoid confusion, it's important to know the terms for the individual parts of the workout. Here they are again, from the smallest component to the largest. If you ever get confused, use this page as a handy reference.

- *Concentric contraction:* a shortening of the muscle

- *Eccentric contraction:* a lengthening of the muscle

- *Exercise:* one movement and countermovement, usually involving a concentric contraction and eccentric contraction

- *Repetition:* the number of times you do a particular exercise without stopping

- *Set:* one complete group of repetitions; the standard set is 15 to 20 reps

- *Round:* a full set of all the different exercises in your training session

For instance, my basic workout is three exercises, each of which involves an important concentric contraction and eccentric contraction: the shoulder press, triceps extension, and biceps curl. Fifteen repetitions (reps) of one exercise make a set. When you've done a set of each exercise, you've completed a round. Three to five rounds constitute a workout.

to keep challenging the muscle with heavier weights or more repetitions.

Let's define some weight-lifting terms right now, before we go any further.

The "biceps curl" is an exercise. The number of times you do a particular exercise in a row is called repetitions, so when you do fifteen biceps curls in a row, we say that you've done fifteen repetitions (or "reps") of the exercise. Those fifteen repetitions of that exercise are called a set. When you've done fifteen reps of biceps curls and fifteen reps of triceps extensions, you've done two sets, one set of biceps and one set of triceps. When you do a number of sets of different kinds of exercises in a planned sequence, it's called a round. Rounds mean a combination of anything from two to five exercises. So if you were to do a set of shoulder presses, a set of triceps extensions, and a set of biceps curls, you'd have done a round of exercises for the upper arms.

I recommend that you do between two and five rounds every time you work out. That's the way you'll see the best results.

Now that you know how the muscles in your arms work, let's talk a little about how we can get the muscles in your mind up to the challenge of changing your body.

chapter five

GET INTO THE GROOVE

I TRAIN PEOPLE in a lot of gyms in and around New York City. Every once in a while, someone who works out in one of those gyms will approach me, complaining that they've hit a plateau in their workout. They see the terrific results that my clients are getting, and they want to know what they're doing wrong.

I know exactly what they're doing wrong, and the problem isn't with their training technique; it starts before they even lace up their sneakers. The problem is their attitude. These people have great intentions, but their concentration and focus just aren't there. They come to the gym to hang out, not to work out.

That's not to say that they're not exercising while they're there, but they're not driven in their purpose and totally dedicated to changing their bodies. They're catching up on the news with CNN while they work on their biceps, laughing at a *Simpsons* rerun while they're on the exercise bike, chatting with a friend while they run on the treadmill. They approach their workouts like an activity or a social event, not like exercise.

You can't get anywhere unless you're prepared to dedicate yourself single-mindedly to what you're doing. It is incredibly important to distinguish between exercise and activity. Walking to work a couple of times a week is better for you than taking the bus, but it's not really exercise. There's a completely different vibration to a real workout, and it has to do with the *quality* of the energy and the focus that you bring to it.

Professional athletes know the power of that concentration. One of my clients was surprised when I started his workout by bringing him over to the television set. We watched as a talented young golfer teed up and prepared to take his shot. Although he was completely still, the mental and emotional energy he was putting out was palpable, and absolutely ferocious in its intensity. His focus created a screen around him that seemed absolutely impenetrable. Just by looking at him, you could tell that he was completely immersed in his own universe, and in that universe, there were no cameras, no coughing onlookers, no birds in the trees, no hunger pangs, no love-life problems—nothing but a man and a club and a ball. I clicked off the set, turned to my client, and told him: "That's the kind of energy and attention that I want you to bring to every set, every rep of your workout today."

I like to call this single-minded focus the "approach," because the way you *approach* your workout informs every level of it. It determines the degree of determination, concentration, and commitment that you will bring to the extremely difficult and rewarding task of changing your body. As far as I'm concerned, your approach is by far the most important ingredient in your new fitness regime. *You cannot change your body if your approach is weak.*

How do you get into that completely concentrated mind-set? You have to make an emotional commitment to your workouts. Eventually, your approach will come as naturally to you as every other part of your workout, but until it is, you may have to act a little—or a lot. Here are some tips that may help.

WATCH THE EXPERTS
Watch professional athletes to see how they build their pregame or precompetition attention. Pay atten-

tion to their body language, their stance, their facial expression, how they move. Notice the kind of attention they're giving to every part of their body. Notice that they are not involved in just a physical activity, but an emotional event.

Successful athletes don't offer excuses. Their focus is on results, and that means that they're out there training, rain or shine, regardless of what's going on in their lives. No matter how unathletic or out of shape you are, it will be extremely helpful to you if you act as if you are already a great athlete. In fact, I have many of my clients say in a convincing tone "I am a great athlete" repeatedly throughout their workouts. You may laugh and feel silly at first, but keep it up and it *will* have a positive impact on your workouts.

DRESS
You certainly don't need designer threads to start a weight-training program, but your clothes and footwear should be comfortable and fit well. You don't need to be wearing skintight spandex, but your clothing should follow your body closely enough that you can see your form and your posture in the mirror. If you don't feel like shopping, cut the sleeves of some old T-shirts or sweatshirts. The muscles you're working should always be exposed.

Clothes tell us how to think about ourselves. When you're dressed up to go out for dinner, you feel differently about yourself, and that manifests itself in the way you behave. You move differently. You sit differently. You might be more likely to flirt. When you put on an old, paint-splattered T-shirt to attack the filthy shelves in the garage, you're sending another message to yourself: "There's no rest for the wicked or squeamish, buddy—it's time to get down and dirty out there."

If you dress differently when you exercise than you do in your normal life (when you're walking the dog, making dinner, or watching movies on Sunday night), you are sending yourself a message. You're saying "Okay, now's the time to think about biceps, triceps, and reps, not about that load of unfolded laundry or the fallout from that fight with my boss. This is *my* time, and I choose to use it by concentrating on changing my body."

MUSIC

As you may have gathered by now, I'm not a big fan of the televisions that you find hanging from the ceiling of nearly every gym. I'm also not a fan of that guy who's talking on his hands-free cell phone while he walks on the treadmill, or that woman reading *Cosmo* on the stationary bike. These people are distracted from their immediate purpose.

One "distraction" that I have found to have the opposite effect is music. Music can help to motivate, inspire, and maintain a proper approach.

Everyone knows that music can help to heighten our emotional state. If you've ever waited to be alone in the house before putting on a favorite song really loud and dancing your heart out, you know the semi-meditative energy that the right music can bring. Boxers often enter the ring to a favorite adrenaline-raising song, and a lot of professional sports teams get fired up by listening to an inspirational song together before they compete. The right music can get the blood pumping and help you to get into the "zone."

Listening to music throughout your workout can help to keep your energy lifted and focused. This is a practical prescription, too—if you're working out to a regular beat, you're more likely to give the same amount of time to the concentric (muscle shortening) and eccentric (muscle lengthening) parts of the movement, and it may help to regulate your breathing.

It doesn't matter if you're listening on a sound system or on a Sports Walkman (to me, anyway—it might matter to your neighbors). It doesn't matter what type of music you listen to, either. One of my clients loves to run to classical music; another client's kids make fun of her because only the heaviest club music gets her heart beating fast.

Most people find that they want something relatively high-energy, so dance music might be a good place to start. You'll also want something with a relatively consistent tempo. Most commercially released albums have songs at a variety of speeds, but you may find that a ballad kills your buzz (or maybe it inspires you more than the harder stuff). You may want to invest in a special workout tape, or take an hour to make a mix tape of all your favorite songs. Have fun with it!

I don't mean to suggest that music is necessary, merely that it can be a useful aid when you're getting into the zone. You may find that it's easier for you to get meditative and fully concentrated in silence. Work out the way that works best for you.

DEVELOP A ROUTINE

A routine can be very helpful in developing your approach, especially as you begin training. Knowing that you've set aside time for your workouts automatically moves exercise to a higher level of priority in your life, and enables you to prepare for your workout mentally.

A number of the people I know work out immediately upon waking up. They get out of bed, wash their faces and brush their teeth, then head off to the gym. Why? Because the early morning is an easy time to block off. It's a time that's separate from the rest of the day and the demands that too often get in the way of looking after ourselves. Sometimes it's hard to get out of the office at the end of the day, and sometimes it's hard to motivate—everyone's tired after a long day. Working out first thing in the morning is a great way to wake up, during a time that's not likely to be taken up by your family or work. It's also a fantastic way to set a tone for the day. Many of my clients tell me that an early-morning workout makes them feel stronger and more confident throughout the day, giving them a sense of accomplishment. That feeling helps them to make healthier choices, especially about food, and is the best inspiration for them to get up and do it again the next morning.

The early mornings aren't good for everybody, though, and it doesn't really matter when you train—as long as you do it. No matter what time you train, you have to take the negotiation out of your workouts. Training isn't something you do when you *feel* like it or when you have extra time or energy. It's something you do on a regular basis because it's a priority for you. You need to think, "It's Wednesday at six P.M., so I'm at the gym—because I'm *always* at the gym Wednesday at six P.M." In fact, the most important workouts (and, as you'll discover, the ones that give you the most satisfaction) are the ones you do when you *don't* feel like it.

If you can't work out at the same time every day, or the same day every week, then the last act of every workout should be figuring out when your next workout will take place. Make appointments with yourself to work out—and *keep* them. If putting them into your Filofax or Palm Pilot, or onto the family calendar, will make those appointments seem more real to you, then do it! I once listened to a client scheduling a routine dentist appointment on her cell phone. She made the appointment for Friday afternoon, a time when I knew she liked to work out by herself. I called her on it: "If you had an appointment to work out with me on Fridays, you wouldn't have scheduled that dentist's appointment. Why is your own workout less important?" She got what I was saying, called back, and rescheduled her cleaning.

I know that we all have other commitments, other priorities, other things on the to-do list. But you're in control of your life, and you can schedule around your workout appointments if you recognize their importance. You may encounter a little resistance from the other people in your life at first, but stick to your guns; when they understand how much of a priority it is for you (and how little effect their cajoling and whining has), they'll be happy to accommodate you. It doesn't take that long to get into shape! Your friends will understand if you move your weekly dinner date back an hour. Your family will pick up the slack and make their own breakfast if you let them know that you're not available to do it.

Keeping those appointments with yourself is a favor to everyone else in your life, too—when you're healthy and you feel good about yourself, you're a better mom, a better boss, and a better friend. Put your workout first, and soon it'll blend seamlessly into your schedule.

Saying "I don't have time to workout" is the same as saying "I'm not that important." If you can't find at least a half hour to train yourself every day, you should consider making some serious changes in your life.

GOALS

Before I start training someone, I always ask about their goals. As I always say, "If you don't have aims, you're aimless."

It's important that your goals be both realistic and difficult. In other words, you need to set objectives for yourself that push you past what you believe you can do without being so far out of reach that disappointment is inevitable. You need to find the balance between challenging yourself and setting yourself up for failure.

I also think it's important that your goals be fairly

specific. I don't think that goals like "I want to get healthy" are helpful, because they don't really help you to figure out where you're going and what you need to do to get there. What does "getting healthy" mean to you? Does it mean weight loss? Muscle gain? Improved stamina? How will you measure your progress? I like specific, targeted goals better, things like: "I want to be able to do twenty-five full straight-leg push-ups," or "I want to be able to fit back into my prom dress." That way, you'll know when you've achieved them.

I also think it's important to put a pretty specific time frame on your goals, so that you're always working hard toward something. "I want to move up to the next weight class (from a five- to an eight-pound dumbbell, for instance) for all my exercises by the end of next week." If you don't reach your goals, don't beat yourself up about it, but take the opportunity to learn something. What happened? Was your goal unrealistic? Are you training as hard as you can, or letting yourself coast a little? Could you be moving up to the next weight class, increasing reps or sets, or adding another day a week to your program? Adjust your workout and your next set of goals accordingly.

We all have a fuzzy idea of the ways we'd like to improve ourselves. I think language is an important tool in your efforts to change your body, and there's something very powerful about articulating your goals. Write a list of your goals and put them someplace where you'll see them often—in your appointment book, on the refrigerator, on the bathroom mirror, or on the back door. Say them out loud to yourself, especially when you're feeling lazy or disappointed in yourself. Your goals can be a terrific motivator! Think of them as promises you're making to yourself, and visualize how amazing it will feel when you've met them. I once saw a woman muttering something to herself over and over again under her breath as she was approaching the end of a very difficult set. What was it that was inspiring her to push past the pain? "Leather pants, leather pants, leather pants, leather pants."

Share your goals with at least two people who care about you, and ask them to do what they can to support you and these goals. If you're public about your goals, it may help you when you're thinking about slacking off—it's embarrassing to veg out and watch TV when everyone in the room knows you should be in the middle of a set of shoulder presses. You don't want to turn your family into workout cops, but if they know your objectives, they may be able to give you a gentle reminder, or help you to reorganize your schedule in a way that makes getting to the gym a little easier.

Keep in mind that your goals don't have to be

restricted to the way you want your new body to look. If you're serious about this idea that you train the way you live, then your goals should reflect that. "I will say and think only positive and supportive things about myself and my body during my workout" is a terrific goal. "I am committed to working out five times a week, no matter what" is another great goal. Make your goals things that you want to do, as opposed to things that you don't want to do— start framing your thoughts in the positive.

Make aims for your workout—and then go for it! But remember, *don't beat yourself up if you don't make an aim,* as long as you gave it a legitimate effort. In one respect, it doesn't so much matter whether or not you succeed—the amount of effort you expend, and the amount of concentration and intention you bring to the project, is the real goal. You need to commit yourself to working the program to the best of your ability instead of focusing exclusively on what you want to get out of it. In this case, it really is the journey that counts, not the destination—because the destination is a foregone conclusion if you focus your attention closely on your performance during that journey.

I promise you this: If you bring real effort—super effort—to the task of changing your body, you will see amazing results.

TRAINING PARTNER

Another good way to maintain concentration and a focused approach is to work out with a partner. If you find it difficult to motivate yourself on a snowy morning, knowing that someone else is waiting for you might make it easier to roll out of bed and into your sweats. If you tend to let yourself slack off at the end of a set instead of doing the reps you're actually capable of, you may benefit from a friendly nudge.

I say this with one disclaimer: a bad partner is worse than no partner at all, so if you can't find the perfect match, it's not worth it. But if you can find someone who shares your level of commitment to getting into the exercise zone and working hard while you're there, it can be very helpful to work out with someone else. This person doesn't have to be your best friend, or even someone you like very much, as long as their dedication to training matches or exceeds yours.

It's essential that you and your workout partner have some ground rules. First of all, when you're working out, you're working out. This isn't the time to debate resolutions to the situation in the Middle East, recipe-swap, complain about work or spouses, or brag about your kids. This person is your *training* partner, not a talking partner. If you want to catch up afterward, that's fine. That can motivate you to get through your workout. But when you're actually exercising, both of you need to agree that this is the time to devote single-minded attention to changing your body.

It's also not a time to be sensitive. Agree beforehand that you will help each other to maintain good form. Correct and consistent form is an essential part of exercising correctly: if you let your partner make mistakes that compromise the effectiveness of the exercise or might lead to an injury, you're hurting, not helping. A gentle touch in the small of the back can be all it takes to correct a slouch; a finger on an elbow can remind your partner to keep their arms perpendicular to the floor. Don't waste the opportunity: ask your partner to make sure that your form is consistent and correct throughout your workout.

When you're training with someone, it's important for both of you to remember to use positive language when you talk about your workouts. To change your body, you have to change the way you think, and changing the way you talk is the first step. Most of us—women especially—are experts at knocking ourselves down, especially to one another: "I'm sorry; I'm just totally lame today." "Okay, I'll try, but no promises." "My upper body is so pathetic." My clients learn fast that I'm not interested in hearing this stuff, and I think that one of the most important things that I bring to their workouts is constant, calming encouragement—and the insistence that debilitating language and posture are strictly forbidden.

It's genuinely exciting for me to see the way my clients improve, and I tell them so at every opportunity. Get away from your baggage. You are not your history! Every new day, every new workout, gives you the opportunity to reinvent and redefine yourself. Talking yourself down actually makes you weaker, so don't do it! Don't use words like *weak,* or *try,* or the evil *can't.* Silence the voice that says those things out loud, and you'll be one step closer to silencing them in your head.

If you catch yourself thinking negative, debilitating thoughts like "I can't do it" or "it's too hard," snap yourself out of it with an affirmation. Repeat three times "I am a fit and powerful woman" or "I can do anything." Refuse to fall into the language and postures of ordinary life. Act, think, and speak like a great athlete, and you will begin to look like one.

You can't be too encouraging when the sneaker is on the other foot, either. Pay attention to every word you say to your training partner, and make sure everything you say is positive. You might feel a little silly cheerleading, but having someone rooting for you can definitely make that last repetition feel a little lighter. Encourage your partner to push past their limits. If you feel they can crank out another rep or two (or three) without sacrificing their form, tell them so—and then cheer them on as they accomplish it! You can even physically help them through the tough parts—a tap at the bottom of a dumbbell or a steadying hand on a triceps to make sure that their form stays pure may help them push past the pain into another repetition.

Tell your partner your goals, and make sure to ask them what theirs are. One of your "jobs" as a training partner is to informally monitor your partner's progress, and you'll be able to provide specific positive feedback about your buddy's improvement if you know what they're working toward. Remind each other about your goals before you begin, and remind yourselves again while you're working out, especially when energy is flagging. This is an important potential source of support.

Remember: A little healthy competition is the heart and soul of athletic enterprise. Obviously, you don't want to let it get out of control, but if you can harness the positive nature of that competitive edge, then you and your partner can use each other's results to press past the confines of your own capabilities. Get the positive energy working between the two of you: push each other hard, and make sure to celebrate as you start to realize your goals together.

Even the best partner in the world calls in sick every once in a while. Don't let yourself use that as an excuse! You're responsible for changing your body, and it's too important to let anyone else blow it for you. Keep the focus on yourself.

A partner is great, but only if they're a great partner. Working out alone can be a wonderful and meditative experience—and if you need encouragement, you'll have this book to cheer you along!

I hope these tips will put you on the road to mastering a great approach. Like anything, the more you work to master this kind of awareness, the easier it will be to do. This kind of concentration is one of the reasons why exercise is such a good stress reliever. It's a legal and safe "altered state"—and it's a terrific feeling! Don't be surprised if you start to crave it. The only side effects are improved health and well-being.

You're doing something very serious when you exercise: you're changing your body, and with it, your heart and your mind. That's not a joke. It's something to be treated reverentially, every time. Respect yourself and the tremendous efforts you're making. If you approach exercise with that attitude, you'll get the best results.

chapter six

NUTRITION

WORKING OUT ISN'T the only thing you can do to feel and look better. I have many thoughts about nutrition (enough for another book, in fact!), and I'll only get a chance to share a few of them here. I will say this: Changing your eating habits is one of the most effective ways to change your body and improve your health.

The country as a whole is in terrible shape, and it's reflected in our health. More than half of all adult Americans are overweight, and a third of the country can be classified as obese. It's a shocking number, and even worse when you consider that those numbers have been rising steadily since the

Are you overweight?

The Body Mass Index (BMI) is the best way to tell if you're carrying too much weight for your frame. If you don't feel like tackling the simple equation below with a personal calculator, there are lots of BMI calculators on the Internet that will do the math for you. All you have to know is how tall you are and how much you weigh. Here's the formula:

$$[\text{Weight in pounds} \div \text{Height in inches} \div \text{Height in inches}] \times 703 = \text{BMI}$$

Let's take a woman who's 5-foot-10 and weighs 168 pounds. She would divide 168 (pounds) by 70 (inches) by 70 (inches). Then she'd multiply that answer (.0342) by 703, to arrive at a BMI of 24.1.

According to the National Institute of Health, a BMI of less than 18.5 means that you're underweight. You're healthy from 18.5 to 24.9, overweight between 25 and 29.9, and obese over 30. So our test case is within what's recommended for optimal health. Please bear in mind that your BMI is only a guideline. Muscle weighs more than fat, so if you're very muscular, your BMI might be slightly higher than someone who's flabbier but weighs less.

1960s. It's not a surprise that we have some of the highest rates of heart attack, stroke, and diabetes in the world.

I haven't put this here to make you feel bad about yourself. When you're starting any kind of health regimen, it's important to know where you were when you started. How else will you be able to feel good about your results? I do hope that it motivates you to start this training program with an eye toward getting healthy. Your risk of developing health problems skyrockets when you're overweight, especially as you age.

When you're overweight, you're literally carrying extra weight—pounds of inactive tissue. Carrying that extra weight is *hard* on your body. It strains your joints, your back, your neck, and your heart. If a client is twenty pounds overweight, I'll ask them to hold a twenty-pound dumbbell and walk around for two minutes. Twenty pounds is a lot of weight. As they start to fatigue, their posture collapses, and they start to get achy and cranky with me. That's when I take the opportunity to remind them that they're carrying around that much extra weight every single day of their lives! Every time they climb up a flight of stairs, or go for a walk, or even just get up from the couch, they're hauling the equivalent of that twenty-pound dumbbell with them. It's a big wake-up call—a real-life reminder of what they're doing to their bodies by making it haul extra pounds.

Being overweight puts a massive strain on your organs as well. Your body is smarter than you are, and it will try to store fat away from your vital organs. This is why women tend to gain weight first in their thighs and the back of their arms, away from their reproductive organs. Men, who have less going on in their midsection, tend to get a gut. Despite the body's best efforts, though, if you're carrying enough extra weight, those vital organs will be affected. Extra weight slows all of your major body functions down; in fact, experts have confirmed that obesity may actually be more harmful to the health than smoking!

FOOD AS FUEL

Obviously, what you eat affects the way you look. It also affects the way you train. The body is an extremely elegant mechanism. It ingests food and digests it, which means breaking it down into components that it can use as fuel, and excreting what it cannot. The finer the fuel you give it, the better your body will run.

Americans have gotten away from understanding what foods make for good fuel. The results are manifest in our overall poor health, everything from increased rates of obesity and heart disease to diabetes. What happens when you put diesel fuel into a Ford Taurus? It coughs a couple of times and dies. A car can't use the fuel intended for a truck. That's what happens when you eat a Twinkie. Your body has *no idea* what to do with a Twinkie. Instead of turning fuel (food) into components that the body can burn for energy, it experiences mechanical failure. What happens to the Twinkie? It's stored in the body as fat, like a full tank of the wrong kind of gas.

This is why all the calorie counting and fat watching Americans are doing isn't helping our overall waistlines. Ninety percent of what you find in the grocery store isn't even food. All those low-fat, low-calorie food substitutes aren't any better for you than a slice of pizza—at least the pizza has a fighting chance of being recognized and digested by your body. All that other stuff is going the way of the Twinkie—to be stored in your body's circular file as fat until it figures out how to get rid of it.

A friend of mine plays a game at the grocery store. She claims that she can tell what kind of shape people are in just by looking at the contents of their carts. The more packaged the contents—the more conveniently resealable, red dye number 5, Hollywood tie-in, bright, shiny, overpackaged E-Z open containers she sees—the heavier the person is who's checking out. Conversely, a cart filled with fruit and vegetables chosen from the produce aisle tells her that there's someone in good shape at the helm. It's something to do while you're waiting in line, and you'll be startled by how accurate the results are. The next time you're shopping, take a look at the carts around you, and then turn that same unsparing eye on your own shopping. Is there anything in that cart that you'd like to trade in for a few nectarines?

Here's the simple formula: The more easily a food can be digested, the better it is for you. The more processed the food, the harder it is to digest. So the *least* processed, *most* water-rich foods are the ones that are best for you. And the fresher the better—as I've often said, "closest to the vine is divine."

The best part about this way of eating is that it gets you out of some of the food traps that snare overweight Americans. One of the great American dietary myths is about fat. Fat isn't inherently bad for you. In fact, it's a necessary component to your overall health. The brain, cells, and many organs need them to work properly. Not all fats are created equal, though.

There are three kinds of fat. There's unsaturated fat, which is found in plant products, like avocados, beans, nuts, and coconuts. There's saturated fat, which is found in animal products like meat and dairy products. And then there's polyunsaturated fat (also known as trans fat or fake fat), which is found in hydrogenated oils, which is basically plastic bubbles. Unsaturated fat is easily digested by the body. Your body takes what it needs and gets rid of the rest. When your body doesn't have to use so much energy in digestion, it has more energy to devote to your vital functions, including expelling waste materials so you get rid of excess faster. Saturated fat is much harder to digest and has an extremely artery-clogging effect on the body. Polyunsaturated fake fats are totally impossible for the body to digest.

What the body can't digest—use as fuel or excrete—it stores. So when you eat these hard-to-digest saturated and fake fats, you're signing yourself up to carry them with you for a long time. So it doesn't actually matter how much fat you eat, as long as you're eating the right kind. In fact, doctors believe that the right kind of fat, the unsaturated fats found in nuts and seeds, may increase the incidence of "good" cholesterol and reduce your risk of heart disease.

If you're looking to lose weight, "How many calories does this have?" is actually the wrong question to be asking. So is "How many grams of fat?" The right questions are: "How real is this food? How digestible is it by my body? Will my body understand how to use what I'm feeding it? Is this what my body was intended to process as fuel?"

People always say that they can't diet because they get hungry. Of course they're hungry when they're stuffing themselves with fake food! They're denying their bodies the fuel it needs to function properly, and taxing the organs charged with getting rid of waste. Hunger is your body's way of telling you that the gas tank is empty. If you're feeding your body food it can actually use, you won't be hungry at all. If you feel satisfied, you won't need to eat as much. Your body will take the nutrition it craves and it'll easily eliminate the rest, and you will lose weight.

An avocado, for instance, is considered to be a calorie- and fat-rich food. It's very easily digested by the body, though, which can take what it needs and get rid of the rest, so it's not putting a strain on the digestive system. A low-calorie, low-fat cupcake, though, is filled with all kinds of foreign, heavily processed stuff the body can't digest. Look at the labels on some of these products! If you can't pronounce it, you can't digest it. And if you can't digest it, you're going to be wearing it as excess fat on your upper arms.

FRUITS AND VEGETABLES

Here's the only thing you need to know: If your diet consists exclusively of easily digestible plant matter, you will not be fat. It's that simple. There is no such thing as a fat person who eats only fruit, vegetables, nuts, and seeds. That said, I know that you have to have a very high level of commitment to your personal health to cut all other foods out of your diet. But there's a lot of room for improvement, and even a slight change in your eating habits can yield very significant results.

I strongly advise everyone to dramatically increase their fruit and vegetable intake. Many health experts say you should eat nine servings of fruits and vegetables a day, and I think it's a conservative number. These are *real* foods, and should constitute 70 percent (or more) of what you consume over the course of the day. Let me tell you something else: If you're eating more than nine servings of fruits and vegetables a day, you are definitely not going to be complaining about hunger. Fruit and vegetables are high in fiber, which increases your feeling of being full. They're packed with nutrients, and are easily digestible. Increase your fruit and vegetable intake to twelve or thirteen servings a day, and you're going to have a hard time finding room for anything else.

Make sure your fruit is perfectly ripe. If it's underripe, it's harder to digest, and if it's overripe, it's started the fermentation process, which is rotting by any other name. That causes a whole other set of problems. Make sure to eat your fruit on an empty stomach. Fruit is very easily digested by the body, which is one of the reasons it's so good for you. It passes right through the stomach and is digested in the small intestines. If you have other foods in your stomach, the fruit gets trapped and begins to ferment, and you don't want stuff rotting in your stomach. Ideally, you'd go as long as you could into your day, eating only fruit and unsweetened, unpasteurized juice made from fresh fruit.

Why don't people eat more vegetables, since they're so good for your body? I think a lot of the fear and hatred of vegetables in this country come from our early memories of the tortured and abused vegetables we were served (and forced to eat) as children by our well-meaning parents. I made a delicious salad for one of my friends once, with a base of baby spinach leaves. She cleaned her plate, and when we were done, she asked me what kind of greens I'd used. When she found out it was spinach, she was shocked. She had spent her life as a notorious spinach hater—because she thought all spinach had to be that horrible, bitter, mushy, greenish-black defrosted mess that comes out of a box in order to get cooked (further) into oblivion. She had no idea that the deliciously delicate greens we had eaten for lunch were even the same vegetable.

Because food transportation has become so much better in this country than it was, a much wider variety of fruits and vegetables are now available. The days of grocery aisles filled with iceberg lettuce and mealy cold-storage apples are over. You can get truly wonderful produce at regular grocery stores all throughout the country now. Happily, organic foods, which are grown with no chemical interference and pesticides, are growing in availability as well (if you can't get them where you live, look in a health food store or ask your supermarket manager to consider expanding into organic produce). So there's no excuse not to try to expand your fruit and vegetable horizon.

Eat widely, and of many different colors. Be creative. When was the last time you ate kale, Swiss chard, rapini, collard greens, dandelion and beet greens, or arugula? Or even had a salad for a meal? These options can all stand in for Wednesday-night green beans or Sunday lunch's broccoli. Substitute your regular spud with a sweet potato or a yam. Boil an extra one, stick it in the fridge, and eat it the next day cold—try it as a dessert, like fruit. Switch it up, and try some of your favorite cooked foods, like carrots or cauliflower, raw for a change. Collect the funkiest-looking heirloom tomatoes you can find—the striped, the knobby, the flat, the weirdly colored—at your farmer's market and make a salad out of them and some fresh herbs, like basil. Offer to take some of that late-harvest zucchini off a neighbor's hands and then figure out two or three different ways to make it delicious. Taste stuff! Find a squash you've never seen before, or a melon that looks unlike any other melon you've ever seen, take it home, and see what it tastes like!

And you don't want to get me started on fruit, the all-time best dessert and most convenient snack item on the market. What could possibly be more convenient than a piece of fruit? Bananas and oranges and tangerines come with their own hygienic packaging; a cantaloupe comes in its own bowl! Again, hit the farmer's market and buy five different kinds of apples in the fall. Spend the summer experimenting with tropical fruits like mango, papaya, coconut, plantains, and passion fruit. Keep your eye out for organic producers, and reward them with your business!

The secret to eating healthily is to be prepared by having good things to eat on hand at all times. If there's good stuff to eat, you'll eat it. But if the larder is bare of nutritious goodies and filled with garbage instead, you'll eat what's there. It's no harder to grab an apple or a handful of homemade trail mix, made with raw, unsalted nuts and sulfur-free dried fruit, than it is to grab a couple of cookies. You just have to make sure you've got some trail mix prepared and in the house. And you have to make sure that there aren't potato chips and Snackwells there instead.

I believe that eating nothing but raw, unprocessed food is the ultimate way to achieve your goals of a thinner, fitter, more perfectly toned body. If you want to read more about nutrition, look for my book *A Way Out* at my Web site, *www.matthewgrace.com;* it explains these theories in more detail.

The following chart lists recommended foods in descending order, from the very good to the very bad.

BEST

Raw, water-rich fruits
Watermelon, melon, tomatoes, bananas, peaches, pears, apples, berries, plums, melons, mangoes, citrus fruits (oranges, grapefruits, tangerines).

Raw vegetables
Spinach, kale, chard, carrots, lettuces, celery, cauliflower, string beans, green peas, spinach.

Vegetable and fruit juices (not from concentrate)
If you don't have a juicer, you may want to consider investing in one. You probably don't need to, though, since good-quality juice bars are popping up all over the country. Watch out for add-ins—a fresh, unsweetened and unpasteurized all-juice product is your best bet.

Lightly steamed and cooked vegetables

Potato, eggplant, squash, turnip, parsnips, beets, green beans, broccoli, corn.

Some vegetables have to be cooked to be digestible, but the longer they cook the less nutritional value they retain. Steaming vegetables is a good choice—remember that this doesn't mean cooking them until they're wilted and the color is gone. Take green vegetables off the heat as soon as they turn a bright color.

Nuts, seeds, dried fruit

Walnuts, almonds, cashews, pumpkin seeds, Brazil nuts, dates, dried apricots, prunes, raisins.

Make sure to choose raw and unsalted nuts, and make sure that your dried fruit is organic to ensure that it hasn't been dried using a sulfur-based drying process, as sulfur is a poison.

ACCEPTABLE, BUT NOT RECOMMENDED

Whole grains

Brown rice, kasha (buckwheat), barley, quinoa

The more whole the grain, and the more complete its state, the better it is for you.

Products made from whole grains

Cereal made from whole grains (make sure there are no additives, like salt or sugar), whole wheat pasta.

AVOID

Bread

The whiter the bread, the worse it is for you. Make your choices whole wheat or multigrain if possible. Bread contains yeast and salt, neither of which is good for you, so I recommend that you drastically limit your intake.

Salt

Salt makes the blood acidic and will cause you to retain water. I use dulse, a form of seaweed, to add a "salty" flavor to my vegetables. Celery juice also has a high natural sodium content and will impart a salty flavor to soups.

Coffee

Coffee is strongly acidic, and causes your body to retain water, and caffeine is an addictive drug. I really recommend that you avoid it if you can.

THE WORST OF THE WORST

Dairy products

Cheese, milk, sour cream, yogurt.

Because they contain high quantities of an enzyme called casein, dairy products have a clogging, restrictive effect on the lungs and digestive tract. They also are some of the most antibiotic- and steroid-laden products in the modern American diet.

Tofu

I know tofu is a popular health food, but it's a highly processed product, and difficult to digest as a result.

Meat

Chicken, red meat, pork.

If you must have meat, bake or broil it, and eat it with a vegetable-only salad—no bread, pasta, or rice. And if you have to eat meat and fish, it's really worth it to seek out the organic kind. It's more expensive, but I think it's a small price to pay for what you get. Organic farmers are much more careful about the things that matter. They don't use growth hormones, toxic feeds, or antibiotics, and they pay closer attention to what the animal eats.

Refined sugar and caffeine

Caffeine and sugar (or aspartame, a fake chemical compound in the "diet" stuff) do terrible things to your body. Replace sodas and other similar beverages with water or juice.

With this chart in hand, take half an hour and clean out your kitchen, looking at your staples through the prism of your new knowledge about fresh food and digestibility. It'll be very satisfying to get rid of this stuff, and it's a sure sign to the universe and yourself that you mean business! On your next trip to the supermarket, stock up on lots of fruits and vegetables. Every time you see your clean cupboard shelves and produce-filled refrigerator, it will help to keep you on track.

EAT LESS

Contrary to what a lot of the "experts" will tell you, I believe that three meals a day is too much food, and that breakfast is less important than everyone believes. All the longevity studies are showing now that the key to a longer life is less food. Ideally, you'd eat one meal plus a healthy snack, but two to three small meals is acceptable. You'll be amazed how much better your body's performance is when it's out from under the burden of too much food. It may take a few days to adjust, but the results will be worth the short-term sacrifice.

WATER

There's a big movement in the health industry to encourage what I consider to be excessive water consumption. You certainly don't need to choke down eight glasses of water a day if you're getting the majority of your nutrition through water-rich fruits and vegetables, and doing so may put a strain on your kidneys. I'd advise you to drink when—and only when—you're thirsty.

A note about water: Chlorine and fluoride are cancer-causing poisons, and yet they're the chemicals used to "clean" our water supply. It's essential to drink water that's been stripped of these chemicals: either the best bottled water you can find, distilled water, or water that's been cleaned by a water filtration system. There are a number of inexpensive versions of these filtration systems on the market, like the Brita water system, which is a refillable pitcher that can be kept in the refrigerator. If you're seriously committed to good health, you may want to invest in a filtration system for your home. You have to wash your fruits and veggies, and there's no reason not to use the cleanest water possible.

Following a diet of foods that are easier to digest is more than just a way to lose weight—it's a way to better health. I personally believe that if people in this country moved away from processed foods, we'd have *much* fewer instances of disease and increased longevity.

EATING BEFORE YOU WORK OUT

I know a lot of trainers believe that you should eat a small meal an hour or so before you work out, "for energy." I believe the opposite: if you're looking to lose weight or burn fat, you should work out on an empty stomach.

Here's the logic behind this: The body burns carbohydrates and complex sugars first, then fat, then protein, or muscle tissue (this is called ketosis, and it's what happens when you starve—or go on one of those high-protein, no-carbohydrate diets). Your body will always look for immediately accessible sources of carbohydrates first, so if you eat an apple before you work out, your body will use that energy first. Only when the apple's energy is depleted will your body turn to your fat stores for more energy.

If the point of working out is to burn some fat, then doesn't it make sense to cut to the chase and start doing that immediately, instead of wasting time burning the apple?

It's easy to work out on an empty stomach if it's the first thing you do in the morning, but schedules are busy, and mornings may not be the best time to work out for you. You can still make sure there's nothing in your stomach by eating a light, easily digestible meal a couple of hours before you work out. How long you eat before you work out depends on the meal—what and how many different kinds of things you eat. Watermelon will basically be digested in forty-five minutes, whereas a banana might take a little longer. A more complex meal, with a number of different ingredients, might take between three to eight hours. Everyone's body is different; you might learn that you have difficulty digesting some things and no difficulty at all with others. If you pay attention to the way you feel after you've eaten—and a couple of hours after you've eaten—you'll get to know your own system and can make decisions accordingly.

If you absolutely need something in your stomach before you head off to work out, there's nothing wrong with a little diluted, unsweetened, unpasteurized, fresh fruit juice. It's very rare to experience hunger during a serious workout—when you're working hard, the body diverts all of its available energy away from the digestive system to the muscles. If you can just get a little ways into your workout, you won't be distracted by hunger pangs. Do stay hydrated throughout your workout by drinking water to satisfy thirst.

EATING AFTER YOU WORK OUT

For maximum results, you should wait twenty to thirty minutes after your workout to eat. Many people do get hungry or thirsty after physical activity, so feel free to have a glass of fresh juice or an apple. These options will satisfy your craving without affecting your toning.

I have to say that one of the best things about working out regularly is how good food tastes afterward! Food tastes *amazing* when you're hungry—unfortunately, we live in such a sedentary world that it's hard to really work up a decent appetite when all you're doing is walking from your house to the car to your office and then back to the car. You'll definitely notice an increase in your appetite when you start working out. Go ahead and eat! Your body is telling you that it needs fuel. As long as you feed it food that's good for it, you won't gain weight. And the improved circulation you'll experience from working out helps all parts of your body—including your sense of taste.

So work out on an empty stomach. You'll burn fat and work up a real appetite!

chapter seven

AEROBIC EXERCISE

CARDIO, SHORT FOR cardiovascular exercise (also called aerobic exercise) is the other crucial component in your ten-day blitz toward the toned arms of your dreams.

Cardio is great for your body—and not just the way it looks, either. Aerobic exercise trains your cardiovascular system (your heart and blood vessels) to work more efficiently, pushing nonoxygenated blood to the lungs and oxygenated blood to the cells in the body that need it. Studies have shown that even a moderate amount of cardio can decrease blood pressure, lower cholesterol, promote weight loss, and improve overall mood.

You're doing cardio when your heart rate is elevated. Your target heart rate (the heart rate you want to maintain throughout your workout) is between 50 percent to 75 percent of your maximum heart rate. According to the American Heart Association, your maximum heart rate is the most number of beats your heart can safely beat in a minute. The average maximum heart rate is 220 minus your age. So the maximum heart rate for a thirty-five-year-old woman is 185 beats per minute (bpm). That means that your heart shouldn't beat more than 185 beats a minute (or 30 beats every ten seconds). Her target heart rate is half to three-quarters of that, between 93 and 138 beats a minute (or between 15 and 23 beats every ten seconds).

Here are those equations again:

Maximum heart rate = 220 minus your current age

Target heart rate (low end) =
maximum heart rate multiplied by .5

Target heart rate (high end) =
maximum heart rate multiplied by .75

(The results can be divided by six to discover the number of beats every ten seconds.)

Whatever you do, you want to get your heart rate up for a *minimum* of twenty minutes, and I recommend that you do at least a half hour of cardio a minimum of three times a week if you want to start burning fat. To get in shape quickly, working out every day for ten days will greatly help, and even twice a day won't hurt.

Many gym machines have ways to monitor your heart rate. You can also buy an inexpensive heart-rate monitor at sports stores—the readout is on a watch-like apparatus that you attach to your wrist, and your heart rate is measured by a strap wrapped around your chest. You can also figure out your heart rate the old-fashioned way—by feeling for your pulse, either at your neck or at your wrist—with your fingers, and counting the number of beats you feel. You may want to count for ten seconds and then multiply the number you get by six to come up with the number of beats per minute. One of my clients has a good trick: she just checks the pulse at her throat. If she can feel it beating loud and strong, she knows that her heart rate is up. It's not an exact science, but it's a good way to get an idea.

Interval training has become very popular in recent years, and with good reason. When you train at intervals, you never stop moving, although the intensity of the exercise varies. You'll work very hard for a short period of time, and then you'll drop the intensity back a couple of degrees, for a working "rest" period. Your heart rate races during the intense activity, but never drops completely during the rest. The intervals can be of the same duration, and you'll do a number of cycles—so you'd really crank up the intensity for three minutes, drop it back for three, crank it up for one or two, drop it back for one or two, and repeat until your half hour is up. This works regardless of the activity you choose.

What kind of aerobic exercise should you do? It depends on what you *like* to do. Obviously, if you regard the cardio portion of your workout as cruel and unusual punishment, you're not going to do it. Like everything else in life, cardiovascular fitness requires consistency and dedication, so pick something you like. Feel free to switch it up, too—you don't have to do the same exercises day after day as long as you can keep your heart rate up doing something else.

I recommend that you choose the aerobic exercise that causes the lowest impact on your joints. That basically means no hopping or jumping—a good rule of thumb is always to have one foot on the floor. Running, for instance, is a fitness favorite for a lot of people, but it can be very harmful for the joints, especially for people who are carrying around a lot of excess weight.

If you belong to a gym, it probably has any number of low-impact options to choose from. Low-impact dancing or aerobics classes are great—*as long as they're low-impact*. Tell the instructor that you want to keep it low and she or he should be able to include modifications if the level goes higher. The stationary bike is a favorite of mine, and the StairMaster and elliptical trainer are also good ways to burn fat (just make sure that you don't experience any pain in your knees on the StairMaster). Swimming is a beautiful thing to do for your body—you can get your heart rate up while you're working every single muscle in the body at the same time as you're taking a whole lot of pressure off your joints. The rhythmic breathing that you do when you swim is good practice for the steady breathing you need to lift weights effectively as well. Using the minitrampoline, or "rebounding," is also a great low-impact exercise.

If you want to take your cardio outside, consider cycling or fast walking in good footwear. There's nothing wrong with working out outside as long as you don't get distracted and lose your approach. Walk the track at your local high school when it's not too crowded, instead of down to the convenience store. This isn't the time to pick up some juice or chat with a neighbor.

The more cardio you do, the more weight you'll lose. Remember: Your heart rate must be up for at least twenty minutes, and preferably for at least half an hour or longer. It's advisable to warm up and cool down for five minutes at either end of your workout. I suggest that you do at least half an hour of cardio a minimum of three times a week, more if you're overweight.

Please don't overtax yourself. Listen to your body! There's a difference between working up a healthy sweat and giving yourself a heart attack. Rome wasn't built in a day, and you can put yourself at risk for serious medical problems if you throw yourself into a new program without adequate preparation. If you've never done cardio before, ease yourself into it, and work up to the full program. You should always be able to speak when you're exercising, and you should never feel faint, light-headed, or dizzy. Please check with your doctor before beginning any exercise program, especially if you're seriously overweight or have a history of health problems.

chapter eight

GETTING STARTED

ONE OF THE best things about starting a weight-training program is that it's simple! No fuss, no muss—it's a very low-maintenance way to get fit. You don't have to go to a gym, or spend money on a complicated machine that will sit in the corner and gather dust.

The only thing you need to start this program are a couple of sets of weights, a mirror, a chair, and this book.

WEIGHTS
I recommend that you start out with three sets of dumbbells—a light, medium, and heavy set. How

heavy the weights are depends on you—your strength and fitness level right now. You may spend the first couple of days working with very light weights, or you may be ready to jump right in and do biceps curls with ten pounds. Most women work with weights between one and twelve pounds. I don't recommend that you go above fifteen unless you're really looking to add some muscle mass.

We'll discuss the way to know whether you're using the right weight for the exercise at greater length a little later, but the basic rule of thumb is: You should be able to do fifteen repetitions with the weight—no more, no less. If it's still easy for you to lift at your tenth rep, it's too light. And if it's so heavy that you find yourself losing form around number eight, then it's too heavy.

Like Goldilocks, you're looking for the one that's "just right," and it may take some doing. Take your time. Keep in mind that the right weight for one exercise might be (and probably will be) the wrong weight for another. You can get free weights in lots of places now, but a sporting-goods supply store will probably be your best bet, if only because they probably won't mind if you crank out a couple of triceps extensions in order to try them out.

I'd recommend that you start out with one set of three-, five-, eight-, and ten-pound dumbbells (a set means that you have two of each). That's a well-rounded beginner's set, and gives you some room to experiment and grow as you improve.

It doesn't really matter what kind of dumbbells you choose. I like the rubber-covered dumbbells, simply because they're easier to handle when your hands start sweating. You may have a choice between dumbbell-size barbells (a bar with a number of weights that you can add or subtract yourself, with a collar that tightens on the bar to keep the weights from slipping), or weights made all of one piece. I recommend the single-piece weights, especially for beginners.

Keep an eye on the weights you're using as you progress. What felt impossibly heavy to you a few weeks ago will feel like nothing in a few more, and you might need to move up the ladder on weight to continue seeing a difference. I bet you won't be complaining too much when you head back to the store for a heavier set of weights to match your newfound upper-body strength. Again, if you progress past fifteen pounds, increase the number of reps so that you don't put on too much muscle mass. This will not be an issue for most, but a good idea to keep in mind.

MIRROR
Those giant mirrors at the gyms aren't there so people can admire the way they look in spandex; they're there

so that people can monitor their form. A mirror is an essential workout tool, and one that I strongly urge you to replicate in your home-gym environment. You don't have to mirror an entire wall; just as long as you can see what your form looks like, you're all set. The kind of full-length mirror we all have on the backs of our closet doors can be bought for well under twenty dollars at a hardware store. I strongly recommend that you keep one accessible for your workouts, and when you're done with it, you can slide it under your bed without any difficulty.

CHAIR

Nothing fancy—you can probably use a dining-room or office chair. It should be sturdy and armless, with a straight back. Ideally, when you're sitting in the chair, your thighs will be parallel to the floor, with your calves at a right angle to both your thighs and the floor. If you can't achieve that angle, you may want to use a telephone book under your feet for some of the exercises.

THINGS TO KEEP IN MIND DURING YOUR WORKOUT

Certain things need to be consistent throughout your workout. Trust me, I'll remind you about all of them when we're actually doing the exercises, but this is a good, detailed introduction to some of the things that make for a great weight-training session.

BREATHING

Proper breathing is fundamental to a good exercise program. Think about it: You can live without food for a long time; you can live without water for a couple of days. But if you can't breathe, you're dead in minutes. Fresh oxygen transport to all the cells in the body isn't negotiable; it's essential. This is true even when we're not working out. Cultivating smooth, even, deep breathing is one of the best things you can do for your overall health.

Check in with yourself periodically over the course of the day, and see what's going on with your breathing. Do you breathe through your mouth? Do you hold your breath when you're going up the stairs? Do you cheat yourself by sipping tiny breaths instead of taking deep ones? When you have an altercation with your boss or your children, does your breath get shallow and fast? This is what happens when we're frightened or threatened in some way, and it triggers a whole lot of other unpleasant, fight-or-flight reactions in our other systems. If you can get (and keep) control of your breath, then you're really in command of your whole body.

Really concentrate on slowing your breathing

down, fully inflating the lungs, and releasing all of the air before you take another breath. Many of us are using such a small percentage of our lung capacity that we're often surprised to learn how deep and wide the lungs actually are when they're fully inflated. I often stand behind a new client and put my hands on their lowest ribs and back, and then encourage them to lift my hands with their breath. They're always surprised how high they can get my hands. You can do this experiment yourself. Take a few long, deep breaths, trying to take in more air with every one. On the final breath, hold it, and try to take in just a little bit more. Can you feel how big your lungs are?

Although I believe in breathing through your nostrils when you're not working out, you'll need to pull a little more oxygen when you're lifting weights, so breathe in and out through your mouth. Take long, deep, even breaths at all times. Exhale when the body is working. Never *ever* hold your breath during an exercise.

POSTURE

If only people knew how important posture is! First of all, good breathing is impossible without proper posture, and as I've explained, good breathing is essential. You can't breathe well if you're hunched over, compressing the lungs and crushing the diaphragm.

Experiment with posture quickly. Stand normally in front of a full-length mirror. Check your alignment. Are your shoulders at the same height? Are you rounded and collapsed in the front? Are your hips squared to the front or are they uneven and twisted? Where are your feet pointed? What's going on with your lower back?

Now exaggerate your "poor" posture. Let your shoulders round. Drop your chin, slump through your midsection, and allow yourself to really collapse into your lower half. Make a mental note of the way this feels: the strain it puts on your back, and the way it compresses your breathing.

Then plant your feet hip width apart, with your feet parallel and a microbend in the knees (your knees should be slightly soft, not locked in a straight position). Feel that your weight is distributed equally between your two feet. Move your shoulders up and back, squaring them, and pulling your chest up. Let your arms hang naturally by your side. Tuck your tailbone, so your back is in a neutral position, and there's a straight line between your heels, your butt, and the top of your head. Gaze at a spot directly in front of you at eye level. Now take a deep breath in. Feel the difference?

Posture isn't only about good breathing. Good alignment is the single most important way to stay injury-free. Assume the "good posture" position again. Now move one of your feet, so that the toe points outward slightly. Do you feel how that subtly changes everything? Suddenly everything's out of whack. Your hips have twisted slightly out of alignment, and you've put strain on all your major joints, including the ankle, the knee, and the lower back. This is why it's so important to stay conscious of your posture throughout your workout. If you tried to lift a weight now, you'd be at a disadvantage and in danger of getting hurt. Moving your foot an inch or two seems like such a small thing, but it can make a real difference.

One of the best ways to stay on top of your posture is to keep checking yourself in the mirror. You should do a posture check at the beginning of every exercise, and you should keep checking on it throughout each rep and all the way through your workout, ensuring that it's as pristine on the fifteenth rep as it was on the first. Your posture will automatically improve if you do this every time you work out. Imagine a series of straight lines across your shoulders and hips. Imagine parallel straight lines governing your thighs and feet. Imagine a straight line connecting the top of your head to the back of your neck to your upper back. As you work out, check those lines to make sure that they stay straight, no matter what.

A final word about posture. Did you notice anything else when you were doing the "good" and "poor" posture exercises? Do them again, and this time notice how different you look when you're standing up straight. It's a major improvement, isn't it? It's one of the first things celebrities learn about looking good, and it's why professional athletes and dancers look so good in street clothes. They're in control of their "body language"—the way their body communicates information about them to the outside world. It's a confidence builder, too. As soon as you get a little length into your spine and push your shoulders back, you look taller, more confident, stronger, and yes, thinner. That's a pretty compelling improvement in itself, isn't it?

PROPER FORM

I cannot emphasize how important it is to do these exercises correctly. At best, doing an exercise wrong will compromise your results. At worst, it can cause you serious injury. Learning and maintaining correct form is the single most important thing you can do to get your desired result.

Proper form is also the only way to make sure that you're improving! If you do the exercise the same way every time, and you're able to do more reps or lift more weights, then you'll *know* you've gotten stronger and more toned. If you're doing the exercise differently every time, one day it'll be easy, and the next day it'll be impossible. That's because, in some cases, you will have been "cheating" by using momentum or other muscles.

One of the real cornerstones of this program is that as you get stronger, you'll have to increase the amount of weight or the number of reps in order to continue to see progress. If your form isn't rock solid and constant, then you won't be able to accurately monitor your progress and tailor the program to suit your changing body.

Certain aspects of proper form pervade every exercise. Here are some of the basics:

1. Never lock out your joints. When you straighten a joint (like your elbow or your knee) as far as it will go, you're "locking it out." It's also called hyperextension, and it puts strain on the joint in question. When you hyperextend, you're putting yourself at serious risk for an injury.

You can train yourself not to lock your joints, but it will take a little mindfulness at first. In a controlled fashion, stand up and push your knees as far back as they can possibly get (just this once!). That's what it means to lock out a joint. Stand up again, and now, instead of locking your knees, preserve a minuscule bend there. This is called a microbend. The joint is still straight, but in a neutral position, with just a slight softening in the joint. A microbend is the safe and correct posture for most standing exercises.

The same is true whenever I call for you to straighten or extend your arm in the exercises. Try it without a weight: straighten your arm, forcing the elbow to hyperextend. Now release it slightly, so that there's still tension on the muscle, but with a microbend in the elbow. This is the correct extended position.

2. Every time you lift a weight, you must initiate the movement from the muscle you're intending to target. In other words, if you're doing a biceps curl, the impetus to move the weight must originate from your biceps. It sounds self-evident, right? But it's not our first impulse, unless we train ourselves to work out this way. Try it once with a light weight, thinking only about getting the weight from one place to another, and then again, really concentrating on making sure that the movement starts and ends with the biceps muscle. Do you see how much more complete and concentrated the second move is? That's the key to getting the most out of every rep.

Remember, "bring it" don't "swing it."

3. Maintain proper posture. I know I sound like a broken record, but proper posture is absolutely critical. Poor posture puts you at risk for injury, compromises your breathing, and has a detrimental effect on your form.

Your shoulders should be back and down, and you must maintain a subtle S-curve in your back so that your chest sticks out slightly. Your chin should be parallel to the floor. If you're standing, your legs should be hip width apart, and the outsides of your feet should be parallel to each other. If you're sitting, your weight should be equally distributed between your sit bones (the bones in your butt you actually sit on), with your feet parallel, legs coming straight out from your hips. Eventually, this correct posture will become second nature; until then, please make a special note of it when you set up for an exercise, and maintain proper posture throughout the set.

4. Never "break" your wrist. A common mistake with beginning weight lifters is to rotate the wrist to help lift the weight. For instance, if the weight is being raised, they will flip the wrist up to accelerate the motion. This flopping of the wrist is not only bad form, it is the leading cause of injury (along with poor posture) among weight lifters, both from strained wrists and from repetitive stress on the wrist joint.

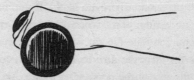

The key to avoiding these injuries is to keep the wrist still (known as "unbroken") throughout the exercise. In the starting position, the wrist should be flat, which means the upper part of the hand and the lower part of the arm should come as close as possible to forming a straight line (see illustration). This position must be retained throughout the exercise. Even when the exercise calls for a change in hand position, this is accomplished by rotating the entire lower arm, not the wrist.

Maintaining a flat wrist will keep the pressure on the targeted muscle, and keep you from strains and soreness down the road.

5. Use the same weight, and do the same number of repetitions, for each arm. You may feel as though one side of your body is stronger than the other. Chances are good that you're right. You want to work toward a symmetrical body, though, so you must use the same amount of weight for the same number of repetitions on each side. Your dominant side (usually the hand you write with) will probably be the stronger one when you begin. If you find one arm failing earlier, don't worry about it. Drop that weight and continue the set with the stronger arm, then use the stronger arm to help the weaker one through the rest of the reps. After a week or two of working out, your sides should begin to even out.

6. Use the right weight for the exercise. You'll notice that I haven't specified how heavy the weights should be for each exercise. There's a good reason for that: everyone's different! We're all working with different body types as well as different levels of natural strength and fitness. So what may be a real strain for your workout partner might be a cakewalk for you, and vice versa. We're strong in different parts of our bodies, depending on how we're built and the kind of activity we favor. Someone with underdeveloped biceps might have extraordinary shoulder strength, for instance.

How will you know what weight is right for you? There's only one way to know, and that's to do a set of exercises to find out. Start light. Avoiding injury should be your first priority when you're starting an exercise regime: *no one ever got hurt by using a weight that was too light for them.*

By the eighth repetition, you should feel a slight burn or fatigue in the muscle you're working. If you're just cruising along happily, that weight is too light for you. If you're working out with weights that are too light, *you will not see progress*. You probably will find yourself going up a weight class or two over the course of the ten days, but if you don't, don't be discouraged. Everyone's body is different. What's important is that you're working hard and pushing yourself.

7. Remember those super-important negative reps. Don't let yourself relax when you're returning the weight to the ready position or you'll be working out inefficiently and wasting your own time. Concentrate on every aspect of the movement equally and control the weight the entire time.

Remember, that burn you feel is just the beginning of the work—you want to be able to do another seven reps, fully overloading the muscle and really getting the most out of your workout. As you get stronger, monitor the burn. If you're not feeling it by the eighth rep, you're ready to move up to a heavier weight. If you can't get through the fifteen with a heavier weight, take a minibreak (no more than five seconds) when you start to fail and then try to complete the set.

For instance, you're barely about to do the twelfth rep and the thirteenth is not going to happen. Rest for a count of five, without putting the weights down, and get three more reps in, instead of giving up. You'll be up to fifteen consecutive reps within the week.

When you find the right weight, make a note next to the exercise so that you'll remember for next time. Leave lots of room for the next weight class—and the next! Make copies of the "My Ten-Day Workout" chart on pages 118–119 and use it as a permanent record of the progress you make.

RESTING BETWEEN SETS

Weight training can be an extremely efficient way to work both your musculature and your cardiovascular system. To make sure you're getting all the benefits from your weight-training workout, you have to work at the right intensity.

That's why the amount of rest that you take—between exercises, and between sets—directly affects the kind of workout you get. If you take the time to really "catch your breath," you're letting your heart rate drop and losing all the advantages that come with elevation. Work through your fatigue and you'll find yourself getting fitter faster—which means that you'll be less tired every time you work out.

As a rule, you should never rest between repetitions—think of each exercise as a single unit of movement. I recommend that you start out with a one-minute rest between rounds (certainly no more than two minutes). This should give you enough time to regulate your breath and set yourself up properly for the next round. Eventually, I'd like you to be able to move immediately from one round to the next without resting at all so that your heart rate stays elevated throughout the workout. It also makes your workout more efficient—if you're not resting, you can be in and out in twenty minutes.

chapter nine

TONED ARMS IN TEN DAYS: THE WORKOUT

YOU HAVE TEN days to get your upper arms in fighting shape. It's not a lot of time, but trust me: you can do a lot in ten days.

The first workout you'll find here is what we call the basic workout. It hits all three of the major muscles in the upper arm in a quick series of easy-to-master, super-effective exercises. Do the basic workout every day for ten days—or forever—and you will notice a major change in your body. I guarantee it.

In the maintenance chapter, you'll also find three add-on workouts. You can "add" these exercises on to your basic workout. You'll still be doing the Basics every day, but as you get stronger and more experienced, you may want to mix it up a little. These exercises work slightly different parts of the three major muscle groups. I've also included some advanced exercises that you can start to add on to the workouts when you find yourself getting stronger.

I'd like to take this opportunity to repeat some terms we'll be using throughout the workout (see box page 32). The "biceps curl" is an exercise. When you do fifteen bicep curls in a row, we say that you've done fifteen repetitions, (or "reps") of the exercise. Those fifteen repetitions of that exercise are called a set. So you've done fifteen reps of biceps curls and fifteen reps of triceps extensions, we say that you've done two sets, one biceps set and one triceps set. When you do a number of sets of different kinds of exercises without resting, we call that a round. So if you were to do a set of shoulder presses, a set of triceps extensions, and a set of biceps curls in succession, you'd have done a round of exercises for the upper arms. The two to five rounds that I recommend you do every time you exercise make up your workout.

Remember that you'll know when you're using the "right" weight for the exercise when you start to feel the burn or fatigue on or after the eighth repetition. Completing your fifteen repetitions should definitely be difficult. If it's too difficult to maintain your form through all fifteen repetitions, it's better to use a heavy weight for ten to twelve repetitions than to drop down to a lighter weight for the fifteen. You'll get those extra three reps in a week or two. Or you can take a minibreak (no more than five seconds) and go for those extra three today.

THE TEN-DAY WORKOUT EXERCISES

These exercises aren't complex or difficult to comprehend, but they may be a little awkward for a beginner. If this is your first time doing the workout, I recommend that you go through all three exercises

---

Here's a checklist before you begin:

- Right Attitude? Check.

- Proper Training Atmosphere? Check.

- Goals? Check.

- Equipment: chair, dumbbells, mirror? Check.

Everything in order? Then let's get started.

---

once without weights so you get accustomed to the movement and ensure your form is correct.

Let's go!

Shoulder Press

Muscle: Deltoid (shoulder)

Equipment: Dumbbells, chair

Setup: Pick up the weights and sit in a chair. Sit up as straight as possible, with your weight evenly distributed between your sit bones. Keep your feet flat on the ground, facing forward, a little wider than shoulder width, with the outside lines of your feet parallel to each other. Imagine a straight line going from your tailbone, straight up your spine, and through the top of your head, right up to the ceiling. Your focus should be straight ahead of you; pick a spot at eye level to look at (if you're working in front of a mirror, you can meet your own eyes).

Ready Position (Fig. A): Bring weights up beside your head so they're in line with your earlobes. Your elbows should be bent at an angle slightly less than ninety degrees so that your hands are slightly inclined toward your head. The palms of your hands should face forward, and the back of the wrists,

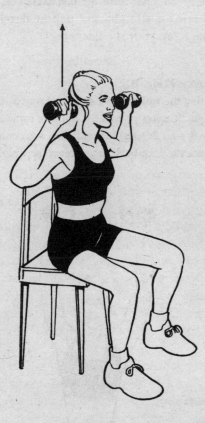

Fig. A

where the hand meets the forearm, should be absolutely flat. As with all the exercises, the wrist should remain straight and unbent throughout the exercise. Keep your shoulders back.

The Exercise (Fig. B):

1. Bring the weights to the ready position. Take that straight line you've created with your spine and tilt it three or four degrees forward. This will counter your tendency to lean back as you press the weights up.

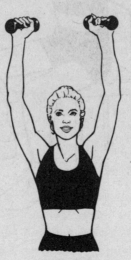

Fig. B

2. With a *smooth* and even movement, drive the hands toward the ceiling, keeping your back straight. Exhale as you push. At the top of the exercise, your arms should be fully extended, but the elbows should not be locked. Hold the weights above your head for one second.

3. Inhale, and bring the weights down *slowly* to the ready position.

4. Do fifteen to twenty repetitions.

What to Watch Out For:

1. It's very tempting to lean back in this exercise. Maintain a slightly forward orientation all the way through the range of motion, and don't arch your back.

2. Your forearms should always be at an angle of a little less than ninety degrees. Your elbows should always stay away from your body.

3. Maintain the correct range of motion. The weights should always return to the height of your earlobes, not above or below them.

4. Control the weights at all times. You lose a lot of the value of the exercise if you just drop your arms back to the ready position. As you inhale, lower the weights slowly and mindfully. You should feel it in the shoulder muscles.

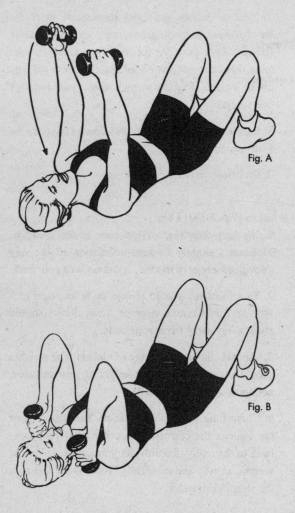

Fig. A

Fig. B

Triceps Extension

Muscle: Triceps

Equipment: Dumbbell

Setup: Lie flat on your back with your knees bent. Your feet should be flat on the floor, hip distance apart from each other. The natural curve of your lower back should be flattened out by the bend in your knees so that your lower back is flush with the ground. Look at the ceiling directly above your head, lengthening your neck, and make sure your head is not tilted back. The dumbbells should be within reach, on either side of your body.

Ready Position (Fig. A): Take the dumbbells in your hands, and straighten your arms toward the ceiling, so that they're perpendicular to the ground and directly over your shoulder joint. The palms of the hands should face inward, toward each other.

Note: For most people, this exercise is more difficult than the other two Basics. Anticipate using a lighter weight for this exercise. Many women start at one or two pounds, so if that's your entry level, don't be embarrassed or take it personally. This is a workout, not a competition.

The Exercise (Fig. B):

1. Inhale and lower the weights *slowly* to the shoulder by bending the elbows. Keep the upper arm, from the elbow to the shoulder, fixed directly above the shoulder joints, with the elbows parallel to each other and pointing toward the ceiling. Don't bounce the weight at the bottom of the exercise; control it throughout the range of motion.

2. Exhale as you evenly drive the weight back up to the ready position, and tilt your hands forward slightly so that the side of the weight nearest the thumb (the back) points slightly upward. You should feel the triceps muscle flex. Hold that flex for a full second before repeating the movement.

3. Do fifteen to twenty repetitions.

Bonus Toning: When you are at the top of the last repetition, and don't feel as if you can do anything more, bring the weight down to the shoulders one last time, as slowly as you possibly can. Try for a count of ten. This is an exaggeration of the "negative rep" that you're doing in every exercise, and it increases the effectiveness of the exercise when you do it really slowly. *By increasing the amount of time you spend working the overloaded muscle, you can substantially improve your results.*

What to Watch Out For:

1. The upper arm *must* stay perfectly still throughout the exercise. Imagine a belt holding your elbows parallel and directly above your shoulder joints, and check your form repeatedly in the mirror. Any movement at all in the upper arm, even a quarter of an inch, will decrease the effectiveness of the exercise.

2. As with all the exercises, you should be working as hard when you bring the weights down as you do when you're driving them up.

Biceps Curls
(also called Quarter Turn Curls)

Muscle: Biceps

Equipment: Dumbbells

Setup: Pick up the dumbbells and stand facing the mirror. Your feet should be parallel to each other, hip distance apart, and there should be a slight bend in your knees. Your shoulders should be back and open, with your chest sticking out slightly, causing a slight arch in your lower back. Your neck should be straight and lengthened, and your gaze focused directly in front of you.

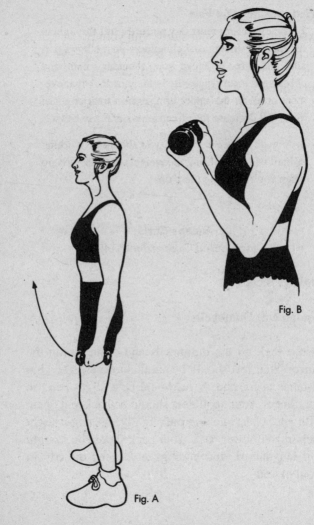

Fig. B

Fig. A

Ready Position (Fig. A): Your arms should be fully extended down by your sides, with your palms facing each other, in toward your body. There should be a microbend in your elbow, so that the arms are straight but not locked.

The Exercise (Fig. B):

1. As you exhale, *slowly* begin to pull the forearms straight up toward the shoulder. The hands should not come all the way up to the shoulder, but should stop at the three-quarter mark, the spot three-quarters of the way between the elbow and the shoulder. Throughout the movement, keep the upper arm and the elbow perfectly still, pinned to the side of the body (or depending on your build directly below your shoulders). As you begin to lift your forearms, gradually turn the wrist so that by the time you reach the quarter point of the movement, your palms are facing the ceiling.

2. Pause at the top, inhale, and begin a slow descent, allowing the muscle to work the entire way down. The hands should remain facing up until near the bottom of the exercise, when you can turn them back to face each other.

3. Do fifteen to twenty repetitions.

Watch Out For:

ep your upper arms close to your body and
keep them still so that you maintain the concentration on the biceps.

2. The entire torso should stay *completely still* during
this exercise, as should the hips. Instead of rocking
back and forth and relying on your body's momentum
to raise the weights, make your biceps do the work.
You must bring it, not swing it! It is very easy to let
your back do most of the work, especially if you're
using too much weight. Watch your reflection closely;
if you see any movement at all in the chest or upper
body, you are diminishing the exercise and increasing
the chance for injury.

3. Make sure your palms are facing up for most of
the exercise. They should only rotate to the side in
the bottom quarter of the movement.

THE TONED ARMS IN TEN DAYS WORKOUT
Now that you're familiar with the exercises, here's
my ten-day plan for a healthier life and a fitter
body—in less than thirty minutes a day! If you don't
believe you're going to get strong and toned, use the
chart on pages 120–121 to monitor your progress and
see the proof for yourself.

These eight tips will take your workout from average to extraordinary, with no extra time or effort. If you need to, clip these rules out and keep them posted in your workout area for motivation and relaxation:

1. Find an appropriate place without distraction. Your mind must be focused on the task at hand.

2. Have a positive attitude and visualize your goals.

3. Use the right weights: you feel the burn at between six to ten reps, no more and no less.

4. Use proper form. Never lock your joints, and always initiate the movement from the target muscle.

5. Maintain proper posture at all times.

6. Breathe *during* the exercise, not after you have completed the motion.

7. Don't forget the negative reps. If you work hard on the way down as well as the way up, you're getting twice the toning for the same amount of motion.

8. Rest as little as possible between sets. This increases the cardio (fat-burning) impact of this workout.

The Toned Arms in Ten Days Workout is three rounds of the three basic exercises, once a day for ten consecutive days. Remember that a round is one set of each exercise, and that a set is fifteen repetitions. If you are using the correct amount of weight (meaning you can *just* complete fifteen repetitions), you *will* see results. For a slightly more intense program, you can do five to eight rounds. I don't recommend doing more than eight rounds, and if you're able to (at the starting level), chances are you're not using sufficient weight.

Each set should take about a minute, which means that each rep should take about four seconds, with no rest between repetitions or sets. Only allow one minute rest between rounds. Your total workout time will be about twenty minutes each day, which is why this workout is so great! Everyone can find twenty minutes a day to start getting healthy and in shape.

If you have some extra time or energy, check out the chapter on stretching (page 175). You may want to incorporate some stretches before and after you train to ensure your body is loose and limber—but make sure it's not at the expense of your workout.

For best results, supplement your workout with my ten-day nutrition plan on page 115.

THE TEN-DAY NUTRITION PLAN

For optimum results, you should follow the guidelines of this ten-day nutrition plan as well. As with the exercise regimen, I believe that once you've adopted this healthier lifestyle, you'll be so pleased with the way you look and feel that you won't want to go back. Here are the guidelines to follow for the next ten days:

- Fifty percent of your diet should consist of water-rich, uncooked fruits and vegetables.

- Fruit or unpasteurized, unsweetened fruit juice only before noon. No cooked or processed food or drink. Ideally, you'd stretch this out as far into the day as possible.

- Eat fewer meals. If you usually eat three meals a day, bring it down to two with several light snacks.

- Out of the ten days, six dinners should be "salad only." Any kind of raw fruit or vegetable is acceptable on these salads: I often use cucumber, tomatoes, carrots, avocados, raw corn and peas, pears, apples, raisins, nuts, and sprouts on mine.

- No matter what you're eating for dinner, it should start with a big salad composed of raw fruits and vegetables.

- Never eat until you're full, and remember, *it takes twenty minutes for the brain to get the message that the body has eaten.* Slow down, putting your fork down between bites, and check in with yourself at the meal's midway point. You may discover that you've already had enough.

- No foods containing preservatives.

- No fried foods.

- No refined sugars. If you're craving sweets, have a piece of naturally sweet fruit, such as a date or fig.

- No alcohol.

After ten days of these lifestyle changes, you may notice that you've detoxed a bit. Your hair will have more shine, your skin will look clearer, and although you're eating less, you're feeling considerably more energetic. You can eat like this forever—you *should* eat like this forever! Keep going.

FREQUENTLY ASKED QUESTIONS
Here are a couple of common questions I've fielded from people just starting the Toned Arms in Ten Days Workout. We've discussed most of these issues elsewhere in the book, but I thought it might be helpful to reiterate them here, right where you need them.

Is it okay to work out every day?
Most people don't like to work out every day; in fact, working out four or five times a week will increase your strength and provide you with some off days to break up the monotony. But this is a crash course to get you toned fast, so for the first ten days every day is important.

There is no truth to the rumor that working out every day will hurt you or will decrease your toning by not allowing the muscles time to rest and heal. Twenty minutes a day, every day, will tone you fast. Ballerinas work out their muscles every day for much longer, and they have some of the most toned bodies on the planet.

What if one of my arms is stronger than the other?
Don't worry about it—it's normal. Work out with the same amount of weight for both arms, and try to do the same number of reps on both sides. If you find yourself failing faster on the weaker side, finish the set with your stronger arm, put that weight down, and then use that arm to help or guide the weaker arm through as many reps as possible. Your arms will be much more balanced by the end of your ten-day workout.

What if I can't make fifteen reps during later rounds?
That's okay, too—remember that you only want to keep working as long as you can maintain form. That

said, do as many reps as you can in those later sets, because those are the ones that will really change your body. If you can't make the full fifteen reps, you have a couple of options. You can take a minibreak (five seconds) to let the muscle recuperate a little, and then complete the set. If a rest isn't enough, and the muscle is really failing, then just do as many as you can. You'll build up to a full set in a short period of time.

What if I get too tired to go on?

Same as above. Although working without resting is ideal, it's better to rest and finish your rounds than to quit midway through because you're tired. If you need to take a five-second minibreak between reps, that's fine. And if you need to take a three-minute break between rounds, go ahead. Just keep that rest time to a minimum, and maintain your focus so that you're motivated for your next round.

What if I'm sore on the second or third day?

Again, this is natural. You *should* feel something— that's your muscles changing, the result of all your hard work. The best cure for sore muscles is to work them, so don't skip your workout. Don't go backward in terms of weight, either—stick with the same weights that made you sore. If you have to do two or three less repetitions one day, that's not the end of the world. Just make sure you're back up to the full fifteen in a day or two.

How soon should I move up to the next weight class?
There's no cookie-cutter answer to this question. Everyone is different, and while I do encourage you to continue to challenge yourself, it's more important that you pay attention to your body and focus on keeping yourself injury-free than to stick to some kind of arbitrary schedule. If you aren't feeling a burn by the eighth rep, it's time to go to the next set of weights. If you are feeling that burn, then you're using the right weights for the exercise. Continue to use that class of weights for as long as you feel that burn.

You can also move up in weights for your first round or two, then go back down in weight for the last few rounds.

If you're training every day with intensity, you're going to improve quickly, and many people will find that they move into the next weight class over the course of the ten-day workout. Don't beat yourself up if you don't, or if you increase the weight for one exercise and not for another. Continue to train properly and improvement will follow.

My Ten-Day Workout

	Day 1	Day 2	Day 3	Day 4
Start time:				
Finish time:				
Rounds:				
Shoulder Press:				
Weight				
Reps Round 1				
Reps Round 2				
Reps Round 3				
Reps Round 4				
Reps Round 5				
Triceps Extension:				
Weight				
Reps Round 1				
Reps Round 2				
Reps Round 3				
Reps Round 4				
Reps Round 5				
Biceps Curls:				
Weight				
Reps Round 1				
Reps Round 2				
Reps Round 3				
Reps Round 4				
Reps Round 5				
Cardio Exercise:				
Type				
Length				

Day 5	Day 6	Day 7	Day 8	Day 9	Day 10

chapter ten

MAINTAINING TONED ARMS

ALTHOUGH THE TITLE of this book implies that this is a short program, I know you're going to be happy with the results you've seen, and will want to continue. Whether you still have a ways to go to reach your goal arms, or you've reached them and want to keep them looking their best, the program can be modified to fit your particular needs.

In this chapter, you'll find three sets of add-on workouts. The Basics will get you into terrific shape fast, but as you progress, you may discover that your workout is getting a little stale. It's a good thing to keep your body guessing sometimes. Throwing some new moves into the mix may also prevent you from getting bored.

Remember, it is perfectly fine to stick with the three basic exercises after the first ten days. In fact, I suggest you stick with the Basics for at least a month. After that, you should be toned and experienced enough to add a few different exercises into your routine, or even an entirely different routine whenever you wish. Remember, any exercise is good exercise, so if you wish to continue the Basics for life, that's great! You will always see results, and these exercises will always be beneficial for your health and shape.

The same rules apply to the add-on workouts as with the Basics. If you're looking to see some improvement, I'd suggest that you just keep going, adding weight and repetitions as you improve. When the weights you're using feel like they're getting lighter (when you can't feel the burn by the eighth rep, and can easily finish fifteen), then it's time to move up. If you really want to see results, add another round or two a couple of times a week, until you've increased your rounds every time you work out. And if you really want to see results, try the drop-set workout recommended in the advanced chapter a couple of times a week.

The Maintenance Program I recommend entails working out five days a week. If you feel that you've reached your goals, and just want to maintain your arms, working out three times a week may be enough. Keep a close eye on your progress—if you feel that you're losing ground, you'll know to add another day or two to your workout schedule. Thankfully, it's much easier to get back in shape than it is to get into it in the first place. It won't take more than a disciplined week to get back to where you were.

In this Maintenance Program, you'll do three rounds of the Basics, adding in two or three sets of one add-on workout. You should never do fewer than three rounds of each exercise. Altogether, you should do a minimum of five rounds, and a maximum of eight. Don't forget to do a minimum of half an hour of cardio every time you work out.

INTENSITY IS EFFECTIVENESS

The goal here is to create an intense and effective workout, and once you've mastered the movements and forms there's no limit to the possibilities.

If your shoulders are responding quickly but your biceps and triceps are behind, do extra rounds of the basic exercises for the weaker muscles after you've completed your first three rounds. Tailor your workout by substituting different exercises from the add-on list on different days. Start pushing for twenty reps in the first two rounds instead of just fifteen. If your shoulders are weak, blast them with five minutes of straight exercise at the end of the workout. You've got experience now, so listen to your body and be your own workout boss.

You're only going to be able to do as many reps as the weakest part of the muscles allows, so pay close attention to the exact place in the movement where your muscle begins to fail. This is known as the "sticking point."

You can strengthen that specific area of the muscle in a few ways. Sometimes just focusing and making a super effort to get through the sticking point is all that is needed. If that doesn't work, you can "intentionally cheat" by using some momentum (as little as possible) to get the weight up, then focusing on the sticking point on the way down. You must focus on this exact area and make an effort to move very slowly through it.

Finally, after you're through with the workout, you can take a lighter weight and "blast" the muscle by doing a very small and controlled range of movement (called minireps) that targets the sticking point (also called the failure zone). This is an incredibly effective way to keep making progress and toning the complete muscle.

MAINTENANCE PROGRAM

ADD-ON SERIES I

Upright Rows

Muscle: Deltoids (shoulders)

Equipment: Dumbbells

Setup: Stand up straight and pick up the dumbbells. Feet are hip width apart, slightly bent at the knees, and the back should be slightly arched, with the shoulders open and back.

Ready Position (Fig. A): Bring the dumbbells together in front of your body, with your arms hanging down, elbows slightly bent. Your palms are facing your body.

The Exercise (Fig. B):
1. Keeping the weights three to six inches from the body, exhale and bend your elbows slowly so that the weights come straight up in front of your body and stop right underneath your chin. The hands and the wrists should be slightly lower than the elbows throughout the exercise.

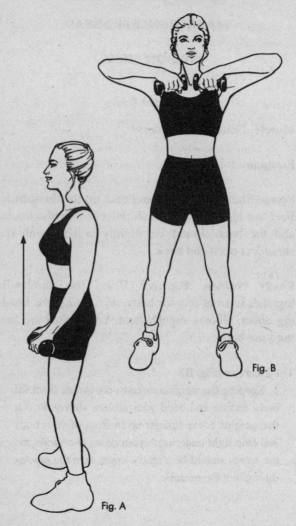

Fig. B

Fig. A

2. Inhale and lower the weights *slowly* to the starting position.

3. Fifteen to twenty repetitions.

What to Watch Out For:

1. Raise the weights smoothly and simultaneously.

2. Keep the hands in line with each other by imagining that the dumbbells are actually a bar that you're raising. The elbows should lead the way and must always be two or three inches higher than the hands.

Single-Arm Triceps Extensions

Muscle: Triceps

Equipment: Dumbbells, chair

Setup: Sit in a sturdy chair in front of the mirror, with your weight evenly distributed between the sit bones. Feet are parallel to each other, and slightly wider than hip width apart. There should be a slight S-curve in the back, and the focus should be forward.

Ready Position (Fig. A): Pick up one dumbbell and extend the arm holding the weight straight up to the ceiling, so that the arm is directly above your shoulder. The palm should face away from you, and the wrist should be in a *completely* straight line with the lower arm. Place the nonworking hand across your waist so your forearm is across your abdomen.

The Exercise (Fig. B):

1. Inhale and lower the weight behind the head slowly by bending your elbow, so that your forearm comes across behind your head toward the opposite shoulder. Get the weight as close to the shoulder as possible. The upper arm must stay completely still and perpendicular to the ground, with the elbow pointing toward the ceiling.

2. Exhale and drive the weight back up steadily, extending the arm back to the ready position.

3. Repeat for fifteen to twenty reps. Switch arms.

Bonus Toning: The great thing about working out with one arm is that you can use your other arm to "spot" yourself. This can help you keep working longer than you'd be able to ordinarily, because you can give yourself just a tiny bit of help with the weight, enabling you to push yourself through a few extra repetitions.

In this exercise, for instance, take your nonworking arm off your waist, and at the point when you feel yourself unable to complete the lift, very lightly

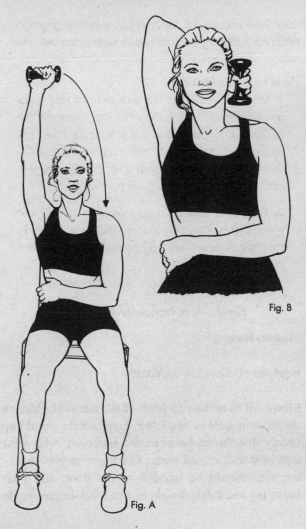

Fig. B

Fig. A

"tap" the bottom of the weight, moving it past the point of difficulty so you can complete the rep.

What to Watch Out For:

1. One of the reasons it's important to keep your nonworking arm across the waist is to counteract the tendency to collapse into one side or the other. It's imperative that you keep your weight evenly distributed on both hipbones, with your shoulders square and facing forward throughout the exercise.

2. The upper arm must stay completely still and perpendicular to the floor. Even slight movement in the upper arm will severely compromise the results you get.

Single-Arm Concentration Curls

Muscle: Biceps

Equipment: Dumbbells, chair

Setup: Sit in a chair in front of the mirror, holding a single dumbbell in one hand. Your weight should be evenly distributed between the hipbones, with your legs bent and spread wide. The thigh on your working side should be parallel to the floor, and your lower leg and thigh should be at a ninety-degree angle to each other. You may have to put a phone book or two underneath your foot to make this angle happen correctly (or you can just get a shorter chair!).

Ready Position (Fig. A): Bend over from the waist with a single dumbbell in your hand. Place the elbow on the inside of the knee, with the back of the arm against the inside of the leg, so that your forearm is hanging straight down along your lower leg. The leg will work as a stabilizing factor to keep the upper arm as still and perpendicular as possible. Your working palm should be facing your body. Put your nonworking hand on the knee on the nonworking side to support yourself. Keep your spine as straight as possible (you will be bent over, but keep your back straight), and look directly at yourself in the mirror or down at your working biceps.

The Exercise (Fig. B):

1. Exhale, and *slowly* begin to raise the weight toward you, without moving the upper arm. You want to turn the wrist slowly as the weight ascends so that the palm is facing the ceiling at the top of the movement. You can come up as far as 90 percent on this exercise and still keep the tension on the biceps.

2. Inhale, lowering the weight slowly to the ready position.

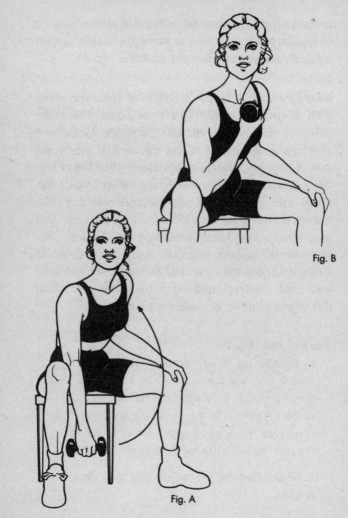

Fig. B

Fig. A

3. Fifteen to twenty repetitions. Switch arms and repeat.

Bonus Toning: In the same way that you can use your nonworking arm to get a couple more reps out of your single-arm triceps extensions, you can "spot" yourself when you're doing this exercise. Take your nonworking arm off your knee and use it to "tap" the back of the hand lightly, to help it through the sticking point. You should be able to squeeze out a few more repetitions by helping yourself along in this way.

What to Watch Out For:
I don't need to tell you to "bring it, don't swing it" again—but I will anyway. This is a terrific toning and strengthening exercise, but you have to stay very alert against cheating, or you'll cheat yourself right out of results! Keep your upper arm pressed firmly against your inner thigh, and make sure that the weight is firmly under your control at all times. Don't rush; go slowly.

ADD-ON SERIES II

Side Lateral Raises

Muscle: Shoulders

Equipment: Dumbbells

Setup: Stand facing the mirror, with the weights in your hands, and your arms at your sides. Feet are parallel to each other and hip width apart, knees are slightly bent, and there is a slight S-curve in the spine. Keep your chest lifted and square (facing directly forward).

Ready Position (Fig. A): Bend your arms at the elbow, and bring the weights straight up in front of you, so that your forearms are at a ninety-degree angle to your body, parallel to the ground. Your upper arms should be straight at your sides and slightly in front of the shoulders.

The Exercise (Fig. B):
1. Exhale as you raise your arms out to the side of your body in a smooth, even motion, *leading with the elbows* and keeping the angle in the elbows constant. The wrists and hands should be slightly lower than the shoulders throughout the exercise. Stop when your

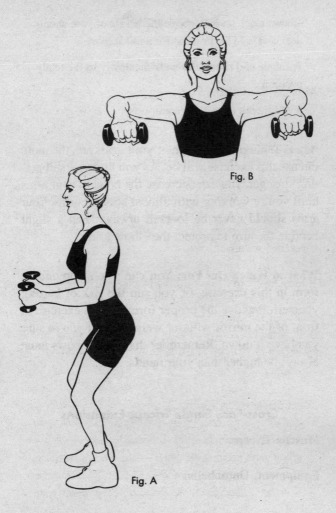

Fig. B

Fig. A

elbows reach an inch above the height of your shoulders, and hold the position for a full second.

2. Inhale and return the weights slowly to the ready position.

3. Do fifteen to twenty repetitions.

Bonus Toning: The straighter your arms are, the more intense this exercise will be. As you find yourself getting stronger, you can decrease the bend in your arms until you're working with almost straight arms. Your arms should never be locked; always keep a slight bend in the arm to protect the elbow joint.

What to Watch Out For: You can't be sloppy about form in this exercise, or you run the risk of hurting yourself. Practice the proper form for this exercise in front of the mirror without weights until you're sure you have it down. Remember that your elbows must always be higher than your hands.

Cross-Face Single Triceps Extensions

Muscle: Triceps

Equipment: Dumbbells

Setup: This is the same position as the triceps extension. Lie flat on your back with your knees bent. Your feet should be flat on the floor, hip distance apart from each other. The natural curve of your lower back should be flattened out by the bend in your knees so that your lower back is flush with the ground. Look at the ceiling directly above your head, lengthening your neck, and make sure your head is not tilted back.

Ready Position (Fig. A): Pick up one dumbbell. Straighten your arm toward the ceiling so that your arm is perpendicular to the ground and positioned directly above the shoulder joint. Turn your head and look at the working arm. For instance, if you're exercising the right arm, turn your head to the right.

The Exercise (Fig. B):
   1. As in the triceps extension, you'll be bending the elbow to bring the weight down without moving the upper arm at all. But instead of bringing the weight straight down to your shoulder, turn your palm to face away from you, inhale, and bring the weight down **across** your face. Gently touch your cheek with the weight (this should provide you with some incentive to control the weight on the way down!).

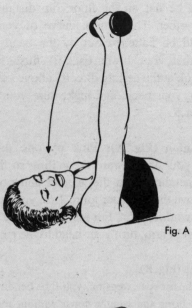

Fig. A

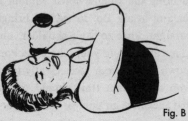

Fig. B

2. Exhale and drive the weight back up to a straight-arm, extended position.

3. Do fifteen to twenty repetitions. Switch arms and repeat.

Bonus Toning: As we know, one of the benefits of working one arm at a time is that you can "spot" yourself, which may allow you to push past your limits and crank out a few more reps, increasing muscle exhaustion (and your results!). Be careful with this one, though—I don't want you dropping the weight on your face!

If you're feeling particularly ambitious and really want your triceps to burn, you can do fifteen to twenty reps on one arm, switch arms, and then switch *again*, continuing alternating sets until the muscle is exhausted. Try to do at least five sets, keeping your heart rate up while you really focus on a single muscle group. If you do this, you may have to decrease the amount of reps you attempt on the second and third consecutive sets. So if you do fifteen reps on the first set, you may want to try twelve on the second and between eight and ten on the third. That's fine; just make sure you do the same number on each side.

Turned-Out Curl

Muscle: Biceps

Equipment: Dumbbell

Setup: The body's position is the same as for the biceps curl. Pick up the dumbbells and stand facing the mirror. Your feet should be parallel to each other, hip distance apart, and there should be a slight bend in your knees. Your shoulders should be back and open, with your chest sticking out slightly, causing a slight arch in your lower back. Your neck should be straight and lengthened, and your gaze focused directly in front of you.

Your arms should be fully extended down by your sides, with your palms facing each other. There should be a microbend in your elbow so that the arms are straight but not locked.

Ready Position (Fig. A): Rotate the arms outward so that the palms and the insides of the elbows face away from the body. This rotation should bring your elbows about six inches away from your body. Make sure that the elbows are completely still and your wrists flat (unbroken) throughout the entire set.

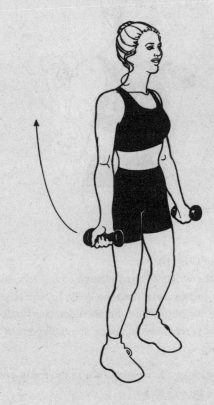

Fig. A

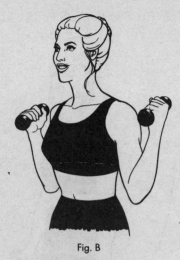

Fig. B

The Exercise (Fig. B):

1. Keep the wrists flat and elbows completely still, about six inches away from the body. Exhale as you move the weight toward the shoulder. Stop before the weight reaches the shoulder, about 80 percent of the way up.

2. Slowly lower the weight down to the ready position, inhaling as you go.

3. Do fifteen to twenty repetitions.

Bonus Toning: Because this particular cu
cult, you can step up results by doing a set o
biceps (quarter-turn) curls immediately after y
ish a set of these turned-out curls.

What to Watch Out For: Make sure that you don't
push your hips forward to help you lift the weight.
Keep the bend in your knees and in your lower back,
and make sure that your upper arms stay still. Initiate
the movement from the biceps—there should be no
movement at all in the elbows.

ADD-ON SERIES III

Front Lateral Raises

Muscle: Deltoid (shoulder)

Equipment: Dumbbells

Setup: Stand facing the mirror, with feet hip distance
apart and knees slightly bent. Your chin should point
straight ahead so that you're looking at yourself in
the mirror, with your shoulders open and back and a
slight S-curve in your back.

Ready Position (Fig. A): Pick up the weights, with your arms hanging down in front of your body, palms facing the body. The dumbbells should be no more than two inches apart. Bend the arms slightly, and move the weights about a foot away from your body. This is the starting and ending position. Tilt your body forward a few degrees, keeping your spine straight and dropping your chin a little bit so that your head and neck are in a straight line with your back.

The Exercise (Fig. B):

1. As you exhale, *slowly* lift your arms directly in front of you until the weights are at the level of the top of your forehead. *Keep the angle in the elbow constant* and the upper body completely still.

2. Lower your arms to the ready position. The weights should always be a foot away from your body.

3. Do fifteen to twenty repetitions.

Bonus Toning: As with the side lateral raises, this exercise becomes more difficult when you straighten the arms. As you get stronger, try decreasing the angle in the elbows until you're eventually working with almost straight arms (always keep a microbend in the arms to protect the elbow joint).

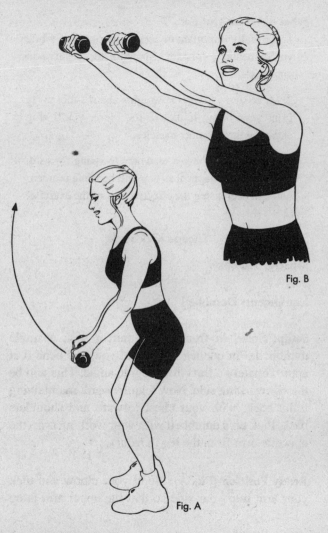

Fig. B

Fig. A

What to Watch Out For:

1. It's really important to keep proper posture while you're bending forward. Maintain the S-curve in your back.

2. Make sure to keep the weights about a foot away from your body. If they're too close, you'll stop engaging the shoulder muscles.

3. The hips will have a tendency to swing forward. Do not let this happen, as you will be using momentum and decreasing the effectiveness of the exercise.

Triceps Kickback

Muscle: Triceps

Equipment: Dumbbell

Setup: Stand in front of the mirror with a single dumbbell. Put one leg in front of you, and bend it at approximately a forty-five-degree angle. This will be the nonworking side. Now lean forward, maintaining a flat back, with your chest forward and shoulders back. Pick up a dumbbell with your working arm (the opposite arm from the leg in front).

Ready Position (Fig. A): Bend your elbow and tuck your arm into your side so that the upper arm is up

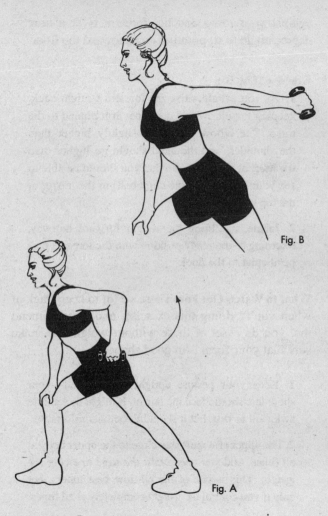

Fig. B

Fig. A

against your torso and the forearm is at a ninety-degree angle to it, pointing down toward the floor.

Exercise (Fig. B):

1. As you exhale, drive the forearm straight back, keeping the elbow and the upper arm pinned to the torso. The elbow should be slightly higher than the shoulder, and the hand should go higher than the level of the elbow, so that you should be able to see your elbow (and the dumbbell) in the mirror at the top of the exercise.

2. Inhale and bring the weight forward halfway, returning to the ready position with the forearm perpendicular to the floor.

What to Watch Out For: There's a lot to keep track of when you're doing this exercise, and I recommend that you do a set of these without weights to make sure that your form is in good shape.

1. Keep your posture upright and aligned—your shoulders should face the mirror. It might feel a little awkward at first, but it shouldn't be uncomfortable.

2. The upper arm must stay close to the upper body at all times, and *you must resist the urge to swing the weight.* This is one of the all-time best toners, but only if you control the weight completely at all times.

150

Hammer Curls

Muscle: Biceps, forearm

Equipment: Dumbbells

Setup: Pick up the dumbbells and stand facing the mirror. Your feet should be parallel to each other, hip distance apart, and there should be a slight bend in your knees. Your shoulders should be back and open, with your chest sticking out slightly, causing a slight arch in your lower back. Your neck should be straight and lengthened, and your gaze focused directly in front of you.

Ready Position (Fig. A): Your arms should be fully extended down by your sides, with your palms facing each other. There should be a microbend in your elbow so that the arms are straight but not locked.

The Exercise (Fig. B):

1. The hammer curl is identical to the regular biceps or quarter-turn curl, but there is no turn of the wrist involved.

2. As you exhale, *slowly* begin to pull the forearms straight up toward the shoulder. The hands should not come all the way up to the shoulder, but should stop at the three-quarter mark, the spot halfway

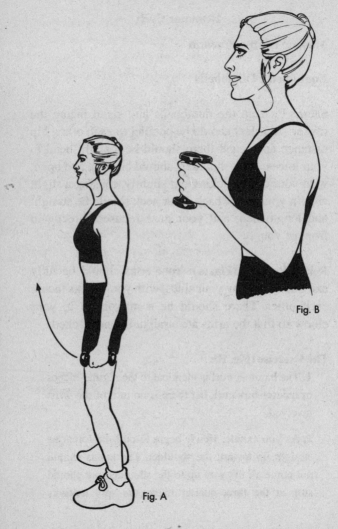

Fig. B

Fig. A

between the elbow and the shoulder. Throughout the movement, keep the upper arm and the elbow perfectly still, pinned to the side of the body. The palms should face each other throughout the exercise.

3. Pause at the top, inhale, and begin a slow descent, allowing the muscle to work the entire way down. The hands should remain facing each other.

4. Do fifteen to twenty repetitions.

What to Watch Out For:

As with all the biceps curls, you can only maintain the concentration on the biceps if you keep your upper arms motionless and close to your body. Keep your tailbone tucked underneath you so that you don't swing your hips forward and lift with your back.

YOUR PERSONAL WORKOUT

Remember: You're going to do at least two rounds of the Basics every day, adding a few sets of one of the Add-ons to mix it up a little. Cycle through these additional workouts—you can do series I on Monday, II on Tuesday, III on Wednesday, and start the whole thing over on Thursday. Or you can create your own Add-ons. Either way, you'll be more likely to stick with the program if you can prevent yourself from getting bored, and I want you to stick with the program—for life!

If there's one thing I'd like you to take away from this book, it's this: You don't need to be a personal trainer—and you don't need to have one—to take control of the way your body looks. You don't have to be a zombie, mindlessly following a program. You'll see better results if you take an active interest in the way your body changes when you change your workout. If you properly learn some basic exercises, you can mix and match those exercises to design your own program, according to what your body needs.

People don't necessarily want to think about how what they do affects their bodies. Their instinct seems to be to turn over the care and feeding of their bodies to a trained professional. But I encourage my clients to actively participate in the shaping of their bodies through the development of their workouts. When they start to get involved, they get addicted. It's a very powerful feeling when you realize that you're directly in control of the way your body looks.

The more you train, the more experienced you will become. With that experience will come a sophisticated knowledge of your own body's unique physiology and the different ways that it reacts to different workouts. Keep track of the changes. Take a good look in the mirror periodically and analyze what you see there. How does your body look and feel? Are you making better progress in one area than another? Are you sore (in a good way) after doing one kind of triceps exercise? Is there one that you love doing?

You may discover, for instance, that you see better results from one exercise than from another. You might learn that your shoulders aren't as strong as you'd like them to be, and you might alter your goals to focus on building that area. You might be looking for a little more definition in a specific area, so you might increase the number of sets or reps you do. One day you might want to experiment with doing rounds of all three triceps exercises, to see what kind of result that gives you.

A lifelong commitment to health and fitness is the best present you can possibly give yourself. Learning an exercise can become an art form. This is not an ordinary task you've taken on. You have the power to shape your body and your life; I've given you the tools, but you are the sculptor.

Congratulations on your choice.

chapter eleven

ADVANCED EXERCISES

WHEN YOU REALLY feel that you've mastered the Basics and the Add-ons provided in the previous chapters, you may want to add some of these (slightly) more advanced moves to your repertoire.

The Push-Up

Push-ups are a classic, and with good reason: they are the perfect upper-body exercise for people who are beginning to move to the next level with their arm strength. Push-ups will tone a number of the muscles in the upper body, especially the triceps, chest, and shoulders. Even better, no equipment is needed:

you're using your body mass and the force of gravity to build your arms. You can do them anywhere, so they're the perfect exercise to remember if you find yourself away from home and your free weights.

A lot of women are really scared of push-ups. It's crazy! I recently trained with a new client, a woman who already had a fair amount of upper-body strength, certainly enough for a set of modified push-ups. When I mentioned, however, that we'd be incorporating a set of push-ups into our workout, her face went totally white. She was completely panicked by the thought of a push-up, although her body was more than up to the challenge. Her reaction proved to me that women really do have a deep-seated fear of this particular exercise. I don't know what it was that traumatized the women of this country—early gym classes, or maybe all those Marine boot-camp movies ("Drop and give me twenty!"), but it's time for that to change.

I'm here to tell you that push-ups don't have to be a punishment. There are many different variations on the classic push-up, with varying degrees of difficulty. Experiment and find the right level for you. Start at the easiest level, and do those until you're strong enough to move up to a more difficult level. Even the easiest push-ups are terrific exercise, and almost everyone who doesn't work out regularly will start at that level.

Half Push-Ups

Muscle: Triceps, Chest, Shoulders

Equipment: None

Setup: To begin, orient yourself so that you can see your entire body from the side in the mirror. Get on your hands and knees.

Ready Position (Fig. A):
Kneel with both knees together. Lean forward so that your hands are on the floor directly underneath your shoulders, supporting your body weight. Spread your fingers wide. The outside of the hands should be parallel to each other: in the correct position, your middle knuckle will be directly under the *center* of your shoulder. Your hips are directly above your knees so that your back forms a flat surface, like a tabletop.

The Exercise (Fig. B):
1. Bend your arms slowly on an inhale. Keeping your knees bent, go down about one quarter of the way to the ground (this is called a "quarter rep"). Keep the body as still as possible throughout the movement.

2. While exhaling, *slowly* push your body back up so that the arms are fully extended.

3. Repeat this "quarter rep" as many times as you are able.

If you don't feel the arms working by your eighth or tenth quarter rep, and are easily able to do fifteen to twenty, then you should increase the difficulty by increasing the range of motion. Go down halfway, instead of stopping at a quarter.

What to Watch Out For: You must make sure that your butt stays directly over your knees, forming a ninety-degree angle with the body. Do not rock forward so that your hips drop and your upper body juts out in front of your hands. This makes the exercise much harder, and does not work out the muscles correctly. The motion must be straight down and straight back up.

If you are able to comfortably go down farther than halfway on this exercise, you are not doing it correctly. If you maintain the correct ninety-degree angle at the waist, it is very awkward to move that far downward.

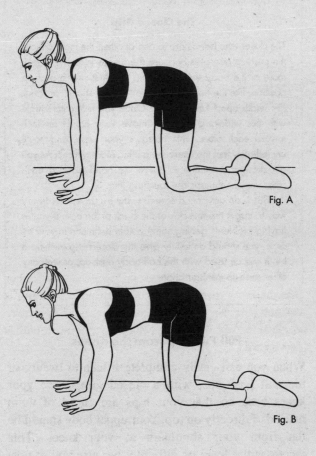

Fig. A

Fig. B

The Closed Grip

The closer your hands are to one another, the more difficult the push-up becomes because the triceps is forced to take more of the body weight. When you first start a push-up position, like the half push-up, your hands should be shoulder width apart (see Fig. A). Once you feel comfortable with this wide-grip push-up, move your hands an inch toward each other. This narrows your base, and you'll immediately feel the exercises getting more difficult. As you get stronger, continue to move the hands toward each other until the thumbs are touching (Fig. B).

This is an advanced exercise, but it's an extraordinary way to target the muscles at the back of the arm. If you're having problems getting some visible definition in your triceps, you should definitely give the closed-grip push-up a try. It can be used with the half-body push-up, or with any other push-up configuration.

Full Push-Up from the Knees

When you can easily complete fifteen to twenty of the half push-ups, with a closed grip, move your knees back so that your hips are ahead of them instead of directly on top. Your upper body should be flat from your shoulders to your knees. This increases the level of difficulty because you're now lifting about 60 percent of your body weight, instead

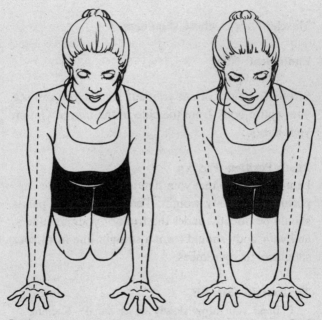

Fig. A   Fig. B

of just the upper part of your body. Use the same arm and hand setup as in the last exercise, but this time go all the way down so that your chest skims (but doesn't touch) the ground.

Muscle: Triceps, chest, shoulders

Equipment: None

Setup: To begin, orient yourself so that you can see your entire body from the side in the mirror. Get on your knees.

Ready Position (Fig. A):
Lean forward so that your hands are on the floor supporting your body weight. The base of your palms should be directly under the front of your shoulders, and your body should form a straight line from your shoulders to your knees.

The Exercise (Fig. B):
   1. Bend your arms slowly on an inhale. Keeping your knees bent, do a quarter rep (go down a quarter of the way), keeping the body as still as possible throughout the movement.

   2. While exhaling, *slowly* push your body back up so that the arms are fully extended.

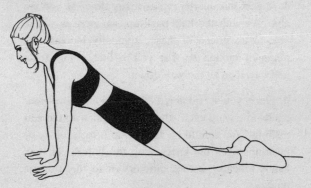

Fig. A

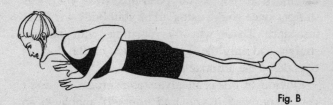

Fig. B

3. Repeat this quarter rep as many times as you are able. As with the half push-up, as soon as you're able to do fifteen of these, gradually increase the range of motion so that you're first going down halfway, then all the way down.

4. Once you've mastered this motion, move your hands in toward each other as you did with the half push-up. You should be able to do fifteen full-body push-ups from the knees with the thumbs of both hands touching before moving on to the ultimate push-up.

The Ultimate Push-Up

It's much harder to do push-ups with your legs straight since you're using all of your body weight as resistance. That's why this position, with the legs straight and only the feet and hands on the floor, is considered the ultimate push-up.

Obviously, this is an advanced exercise, but don't get discouraged if you find yourself unable to do these. Try to do one ultimate push-up every time you work out, and soon you'll surprise yourself. Along those lines, I have an inspirational story that I'd like to share here.

My friend had gotten out of shape after two pregnancies, but she'd begun training and was starting to build some strength and definition. It was hard for her to get to the gym, so she started training at home. Her goal was to be able to do ten full, straight-leg push-ups without a rest, an ambitious goal for someone at her fitness level. On her first try (and her second, and her thirtieth), she face-planted right into the mat. It took her a couple of months of trying and training before she could successfully complete a single push-up.

But she kept at it, and a couple of months later, my newly trim, toned friend walked right up to me at a gym where I train with clients, brimming with pride. Without a word, she dropped and gave me ten. If she can do it, so can you!

I trained another woman, who provides us with a slightly more exaggerated case. When she came to see me, she was forty pounds overweight and had never exercised in her life. She was a very rare case: she did *everything* I told her to do in terms of training every day and changing her eating habits. And her results were extraordinary. I'm astonished myself to report that she can now do two hundred straight-leg push-ups within an hour's workout—including sets of thirty-five reps! She is unrecognizable from the person who began training with me.

Muscle: Triceps, chest, shoulders

Equipment: None

Setup: To begin, orient yourself so that you can see your entire body from the side in the mirror. Get on your hands and knees.

Ready Position (Fig. A):
Kneel with both knees together. Lean forward so that your hands are on the floor supporting your body weight, with your hands wider than shoulder width. The hands should be at or a little higher than the shoulders. If you want an easy way to check how wide your hands should be, lie facedown on the ground and move your hands out until they are directly under your shoulders. The elbow should be at a ninety-degree angle.

Lift your hips and straighten your legs so that your weight is resting equally on the balls of your feet and on your arms, like a tripod. There should be a straight line through your ankles, knees, hips, and shoulders. Imagine that your clothing has exterior seams and line them up.

Note: This position is a good way to build both arm and core body strength. Even if you're not able to lower yourself yet, you can build a lot of strength simply by holding this position for as long as you can.

The Exercise (Fig. B):

1. Bend your arms slowly on an inhale. Do a quarter rep (go down a quarter of the way), keeping the body as still as possible throughout the movement.

2. While exhaling, **slowly** push your body back up so that the arms are almost fully extended.

3. Repeat this quarter rep as many times as you are able. As with the other push-ups we've talked about, as soon as you're able to do fifteen of these, gradually increase the range of motion so that you're going down halfway. Eventually you'll go all the way down, without letting the chest rest on the ground. If you'd like to increase the intensity of these, try another variation: do a combination of full reps, followed by half reps, followed by quarter reps, until you've completely achieved muscle overload.

Bonus Toning: If you find you can't perform a straight-leg push-up, you can increase your strength just by doing negative reps. Just let yourself down slowly all the way to the ground, then start over at the top.

What to Watch Out For:

Keep your body completely straight and aligned. Dropping your hips and collapsing through your midsection is not allowed.

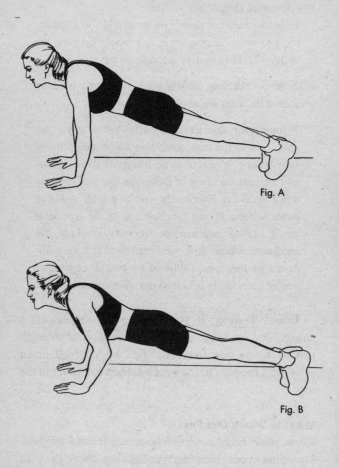

Fig. A

Fig. B

Wrist Rolls

This isn't an advanced exercise, actually. This exercise will tone your forearms and improve your hand strength. It's also very good for strengthening the wrist area, which is helpful if you work on a computer or with your hands.

Muscle: Forearm

Equipment: Dumbbell

Setup: Stand facing the mirror with the dumbbells in hand, feet shoulder width apart, arms at your sides.

Ready Position: Your arms should be down at your side, hands slightly in front of the body, with the palms facing each other, wrists neutral. Your hands should be in a straight line with your forearms.

The Exercise:

1. Keeping your arm perfectly still, curl the hand from the wrist up toward your body as far as it will go.

2. Pause for one second. Reverse the motion, bringing the weight down slowly. Don't stop at the bottom of the exercise, but continue the motion until your palms are facing the floor, so that your knuckles are lifted toward the ceiling.

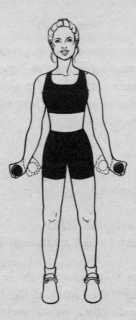

3. Pause for one second and repeat the exercise.

4. You should do at least fifteen full reps on this exercise.

Note: This exercise will exhaust your grip, so it should be done at the end of your workout, after you've worked the other parts of your arm.

Drop Sets

I'd like to take a moment here to talk about drop sets, which are an incredible way to work your muscles into overload. They're a great way to supersize your regular workout, and they're especially effective when you feel you have fallen into a rut and need to wake up your body.

This is a slightly more advanced way to work out. Basically, you're overloading the muscle in one weight class, and when you simply cannot lift the weight for another rep, you "drop down" to a slightly lighter weight and repeat until you've overloaded at that weight class as well.

So if you were doing a drop set of biceps curls, you'd do your first fifteen reps with a ten-pound weight (or whatever weight you're comfortable with). When you start to fail, and you absolutely cannot do another repetition, pick up an eight-pound dumbbell and do the fifteen over again, or as many times as you can. Another way to keep the set going—so that you're working your muscles deep into overload—is to alternate arms, so that your right arm is resting while your left arm works, and the reverse.

You'll notice an immediate difference in your body if you work out this way.

Advanced Drop-Set Workout

If I were to craft the perfect drop-set workout, this would be it:

Do: a set of fifteen straight-leg push-ups
Drop to: a set of fifteen bent-leg push-ups

Do: a set of fifteen biceps curls with the heaviest weight you can handle
Drop to: a set of fifteen biceps curls with a slightly lighter weight.

Do: a set of fifteen shoulder presses with the heaviest weight you can handle
Drop to: a set of fifteen shoulder presses with slightly lighter weights

The drop set doesn't have to stop there. If you want to work your arms until they're exhausted, you can go through your entire set of weights! Start with ten, then drop to eight, and to five—and to three. You'll feel it the next day, I promise.

chapter twelve

STRETCHING

THERE'S STRONG EVIDENCE that by increasing your flexibility, your comfortable range of motion reduces your chance of injury. The way to increase the range of motion in your muscles is by stretching.

I love to stretch, and I think the growing popularity of yoga in this country indicates that everybody else does, too. Stretching may decrease the likelihood of injury, and it certainly increases your overall health, giving you better balance and posture.

You may be wondering why this section doesn't come before the workouts. You're supposed to stretch before you work out, right? Well, as much as I love stretching and think it's important for a well-balanced body and life, I don't think it's an essential step before you work out. Since every exercise involves stretching and flexing the muscles, if you do the exercises with proper form, you'll be fine. So if immediate, fast results are a priority, especially when you're working on a tight schedule, I think your time is best spent actually lifting weights with proper form.

That said, the stretching regimen below will only take a few minutes, so if you have the time to add a "round" of stretching before and after you work out, it certainly won't hurt you.

The kind of stretching you should be doing is called static stretching, where you extend into the stretch and then hold yourself still for a count. You're *not* stretching to the point of pain. You should always feel tension in the muscle, and you should always be working to get a little deeper into the stretch, but you should never bounce to get there, and you should never, ever, *ever* feel pain. I'll say it again: don't bounce. This is called ballistic stretching and can cause injury.

Hold each stretch for a minimum of five deep, slow breaths. Ease yourself deeper into the stretch, and keep breathing! Never hold your breath—your breath is your best friend and an indispensable tool when you're stretching. Use your inhale to correct your form, and use the exhale to move a little deeper into the stretch. Always breathe through your nose, both inhale and exhale.

Remember, stretching shouldn't hurt. If you find that the physical sensation is a little too intense, you can always decrease the stretch a little without destroying the stretch's integrity. Even releasing a fraction of an inch makes a difference, and you're still increasing your flexibility by holding the stretch, even at a lesser intensity.

Women are often very good at stretching their lower body, but I've observed that the upper body is often neglected. The following stretches target the three major muscles in the upper arm that we're targeting in the workouts.

Biceps Stretch (Fig. A)

Extend your arms straight out to the side at shoulder level. Turn your hands up so that the palms are facing out. This will create a slight tension in the arm. Press the heel of your hand out, as if you are pushing on a wall or immovable object with your palm. You should feel the tension in your biceps. This is the basic stretch.

For additional stretching, rotate your hands slowly backward until your fingers are facing down toward the floor. Breathe deeply and hold the position for five seconds, then slowly rotate your hand back to the starting position.

Triceps Stretch (Fig. B)

Lift one arm directly above your head and bend the elbow so that your hand comes between the shoulder blades and the elbow is pointing toward the ceiling. Take your opposite hand and place it on the upper part of the raised arm—not on the elbow joint itself, but just below. Gently put pressure on the upper arm, moving the hand on the stretching side as far down the back as possible. Don't yank the arm, and don't collapse into the right side; keep your shoulders as even as possible.

Breathe deeply and hold for five deep breaths, then repeat on the other side. This exercise also opens the shoulder.

Shoulder Stretch (Fig. C)

Extend the right arm directly in front of you. Wrap the left arm under the upper arm, just above the elbow, and extend the left forearm straight up toward the ceiling so that the right elbow is cradled in the ninety-degree bend in the left arm. Now, using your left forearm, pull the right arm toward your left shoulder. Keep your right arm level and at the same level as the shoulder.

Breathe deeply and hold for five deep breaths, then repeat on the other side. This exercise also opens the triceps muscles.

* * *

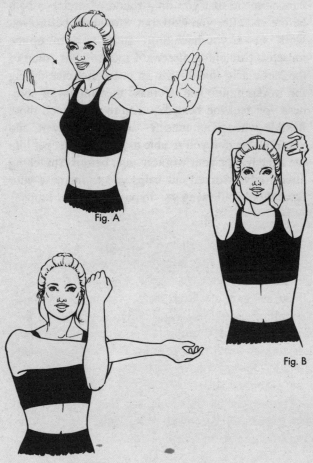

Fig. A

Fig. B

Fig. C

I recommend that you do a round of stretches both before and after you work out. Stretching before you work out—if you have time—helps to warm up the muscles. Stretching afterward redistributes some of the lactic acid that's built up in the muscles during the workout, and can decrease the amount of soreness you feel the next day. You're also much more flexible when your muscles are warm—try it, and you'll notice that you're able to get much deeper into the stretch after your workout than before. Stretching after you've worked out helps you to increase your flexibility by allowing you to push past your limits.

epilogue

TONED ARMS—FOR LIFE!

IF YOU'VE READ every word of this book, you know everything you need to know to change your body. This is a lifetime of training knowledge between covers, and I can tell you—from my own experience and from watching the hundreds of people I've trained in my career—if you work this program, it will work for you.

I'd like you to make a promise to yourself in the form of a commitment to this program. Promise yourself that you are going to give your body everything you've got for ten days. Change the way you think about food. Focus on foods that your body will find easy to digest, and eat less. Keep your training schedule, and bring all of your attention to your workout when you're training. Work as hard as you can—every round, every set, every exercise, every little rep should be the best you can do. Take one day at a time.

Yes, some days you might feel tired, or sick, or sore. And a lifetime of "I can't do it" conditioning might rear its ugly head. You may find yourself getting discouraged. If you feel this way, highlight this sentence: You're better than that, and your body deserves better. Work through it.

You're about to embark on an adventure—and if you don't think that changing your body causes changes in your life, you're wrong! Ask someone who's recovered from a serious illness, or someone who's lost a lot of weight how it feels to regain strength and health. It's my prediction that when you reach the end of the first ten days, you'll look and feel better and stronger. Use that feeling as an incentive to continue. You've spent these ten days taking the first step toward reprogramming the way you think: about time, about food, and about exercise. Make these changes permanent, and set a brand-new set of goals for yourself.

Your journey is just beginning. You're about to do something amazing for yourself. Respect your own efforts, and you will be rewarded with remarkable results.

appendix

LOOKING YOUR BEST

YOU'VE WORKED HARD to get your arms in the best shape possible. But no matter what condition you're in, you can probably benefit from a couple of tips and tricks that will show off the results of all your hard work to best advantage.

- If your arms are thicker than you'd like them to be, you can make them appear thinner by wearing loose (not baggy) sleeves, as opposed to skintight. If you're wearing a sleeveless top, make sure that the straps are wide (wider than spaghetti straps). A straight-cut neck is also flattering, and the lower the neckline the better.

- If your arms are scrawny, and you'd like them to look a little bit better balanced, you'll look good in strapless styles, which show off your shoulders, the biggest part of the arm. Spaghetti straps are good, too. Slightly loose (not baggy) long sleeves are best.

- If you're going to be photographed, watch your posture. You don't want to look uncomfortable or artificial, but standing up straight with your shoulders back will make a real difference in the way you look in the photo. Don't press your upper arms against your torso. Allow them to hang slightly and naturally away from the body. The camera captures only one dimension, and your arms will look bigger if they're mushed against your body. This is an especially good tip for brides.

- Tanned limbs look thinner than pasty-white ones. I know that sun exposure has gotten a bad rap of late, and has been accused of being both dangerous and a cause of premature aging. I disagree with this, and believe that *when taken in moderation*, the sun is not only healthful but necessary. Sunlight gives this planet—and the living organisms on this planet—life. If you'd prefer to stay out of the sun, or can't find the time to catch some rays, don't despair: one of my clients uses a dusting of her facial bronzer to give her arms a little color and definition. Self-tanner also can work wonders.

- I believe that fasting has a beneficial and cleansing effect on the body. If you have an event to go to, and you really want to look your best, drink only water or fresh juices the day before. A single day will improve your appearance, but do not overdo it! One day is the absolute maximum.

- Work out right before your event. After a workout, muscles are usually engorged with blood, and will look firmer and more toned than if you'd worked out much earlier in the day. Working out also boosts your cardiovascular system and can contribute to that coveted "healthy glow."